Survival of the Fit

Survival of the Fit

How Physical Education Ensures Academic Achievement and a Healthy Life

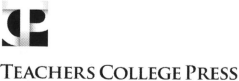

Daniel Fulham O'Neill, MD, EdD

TEACHERS COLLEGE PRESS

TEACHERS COLLEGE | COLUMBIA UNIVERSITY

NEW YORK AND LONDON

Published by Teachers College Press,® 1234 Amsterdam Avenue, New York, NY 10027

Library of Congress Cataloging-in-Publication Data is available at loc.gov

ISBN 978-0-8077-6476-3 (paper)
ISBN 978-0-8077-6477-0 (hardcover)
ISBN 978-0-8077-7927-9 (ebook)

Printed on acid-free paper
Manufactured in the United States of America

For Daniel Joseph "Big Jack" O'Neill,
the little league manager who lost the most games in
St. Hugh–St. Elizabeth baseball history. Yet every child
wanted to be on his team.

And for Jack Foster O'Neill,
born March 24, 2020, in hopes that even without the guidance
of his great-grandfather, he will keep his physical identity.

Lenny: Every being's identity is about play—even an octopus.

Carlos: Can you teach me how to play like an octopus?

Lenny: Yes, as you are very close.

Contents

Acknowledgments

No book is ever written alone. In the case of this book on education, a subject with which everyone has had experience, I have often been surrounded by those with more than just experience, but with actual expertise. This includes most prominently my wife and her three decades in the classroom. The following is just a short list of some of the folks and institutions who helped clarify my thoughts. I truly cannot thank them enough. Also included in this list are my "witnesses" whose words are scattered throughout the text.

Peter Adams, Bard College, Laura and Everett Bennett, Steve Berlack, Michael Berry, Heather Bishop, Leon Botstein, Kathy Boyle, James Carey, Eli Chamberlain, Rick Eccleston, Joseph Ellis, Mark Thomas Evans, Avery Faigenbaum, Shane Finn, Lori and Duane Ford, Sharon Foster, Alexis Gargagliano, Alyssa Greenler, Patricia Hicks, Jeremy Hillger, Meg and Gary Hirshberg, Mark Holoran, Don Hyde, Tony Johnson, Jeff Kauffman, Jerry Knirk, Helen Lyons, Jessica Mayhew, Mary Moriarity, Niall Moyna, Mark Newton, Rebecca Noel, Phil Peck, Corrie Pikul, The Quinn Family, Alison and Bob Ritz, Daniel Rosner, Carole Saltz, Elizabeth Savage, the School of Education at Boston University, the School of Medicine at Stony Brook University, James Stackhouse, Jill and Christopher Ytuarte, and Len Zaichkowski.

Great thanks to my editors Rachel Banks and Brian Ellerbeck for their direction and faith. Thank you to a proper writer, Dorothy Anne Bodman, for her editing and counsel. Thank you Jessica Hoffmann Davis and Ellen Ellis for scraping me off the gym floor more than once. Love and gratitude to my family and friends, most especially my wife, Patricia, and my physical identity Muses: CuChulainn, Mitchell, Lenny, and Carlos.

CHAPTER 1

Our Physical Identities
Inborn, Important, and Impaired

INTRODUCTION: NO STEM WITHOUT FITNESS

America is facing a health crisis of epidemic proportions. By failing to meet basic standards of physical fitness, our children are growing increasingly unhealthy. This affects not only their lifespan but also the quality of that limited life—yet no one is taking action. Thirty percent of American children are overweight, with 20% meeting the criteria for obesity (National Institute of Diabetes and Digestive and Kidney Diseases, 2017). Twenty-five percent of these youngsters have diabetes or prediabetes. Depression, stress, and anxiety are at record levels (Lima et al., 2013). These children will not simply develop illnesses and die at a younger age—like cigarette smokers—they are sick *now*.

Lack of fitness affects not just physical and mental health but everything about young peoples' lives. Study after study shows that poor fitness limits the ability to learn and thus has a huge effect on school performance (Ratey, 2013). We know without a doubt a sedentary child is not assimilating information or thinking to their full potential. In other words, it is hard to be a STEM genius (science, technology, engineering, and math) without fitness. There is a balance that needs to be struck between "nerd" and "jock."

What has brought us to this crisis? To start, children born today can spend their entire lives barely moving. Entertainment in the home simply requires the push of a button. Children do not play outside. They do not make up games with their friends. They do not walk to school. They do not do morning chores. They have less physical education (PE, also known as "gym class") than any American child since school was made compulsory (Cawley, 2005). For those students whose parents have the means to combat their sedentary lifestyle by enrolling them in organized sports, 75% quit by the age of 15 (Merkel, 2013). The vast majority of our children head home after school to lounge inside, gazing at screens and consuming ultra-processed foods. To make matters worse, after they finish high school or college, whether white collar or blue collar, the majority will have jobs in front of yet another computer screen. *Survival of the Fit* makes the argument that unless we change our public schools' PE system, we will not be able to reverse this health epidemic of our own making.

Despite the agricultural, industrial, and technical revolutions that have altered human activities, we are still essentially the same physical beings we were 200,000 years ago. We are hunter-gatherers: designed and programmed to walk or run 9 to 12 miles daily and to eat a huge variety of fresh foods (Kramer & Codding, 1970). Today, fitness experts have set a low bar, asking you to strive for 10,000 steps a day, which is only some 5 miles. Alas, even the 5-milers are a minority, with most folks moving under 1 mile a day as they eat piles of foods filled with sugar, salt, and unpronounceable chemicals. Our bodies are not being used as they were designed. Sadly, this will not change anytime soon, as evolution is a long way from catching up with the marketing of Ronald McDonald and Mark Zuckerberg.

Luckily, all is not lost. Animals, including humans, have what I call a *physical identity*. Physical identity is how we move, how we explore the outdoors, how we respond to nature—*what we do*. Physical identity is our preprogrammed way of relating to the world around us. Children are born as active, curious, motion-loving, imaginative beings with a built-in physical identity—as anyone who had the wrong seat on a flight to Orlando can attest! The desire to run and discover what is around them is an innate aspect of biology, present in all mammals as part of our "primitive" brain genetics. Physical identity also affects the cognitive, or thinking parts of our brain. There is no separating our physical being from our mental and emotional beings (Ratey et al., 2014). If we were to maintain and nurture our youngsters' physical identity, they would continue being the busy, inquisitive people they started as, appreciating and engaging with the natural world around them.

Physical activity, outdoor play, exercise—just *being in motion*—has the potential to give us everything legions of self-help gurus have been searching for: a longer life, academic success, fun, happiness, decreased dementia, the ability to fight off diseases, and more. That does not even consider the sociological benefits, not the least of which are a vibrant workforce, fulfilling relationships, a strong military, and lower health care costs. All of these are potential benefits, yet if we are not making PE and thus physical identity a priority, we are not making basic physical fitness a priority. Without meaningful change, things will only get worse. The good news is that we have the ability to immediately address this crisis: *institute a proper, daily PE program for all students, in all schools.*

Having a physical identity does not necessarily mean being a three-letter sports star, but it does mean needing and seeking movement for physical, mental, and emotional health. Increasingly, only students who identify as "athletes" have hope of maintaining a physical identity. In my 35-year career as a sports medicine surgeon caring for athletes and "nonathletes" (not an identity I recognize, as will be discussed), I have observed an ever-widening divide between these two groups. The days with the vast majority of children being physically active—racing about the neighborhood, choosing sides for a game, simply exploring the outdoors after school—have essentially disappeared.

Although some children get involved with organized sports, by high school the majority end this participation and begin identifying as nonathletes. In my survey of over 100 high school athletic directors across the United States, only a fraction of students played high school sports—yet sports receive 86% of the budget for physical fitness. This means only 14% of the school athletic budget is spent on PE—the only physical activity that most students will participate in. This is happening even though PE remains the one best option to prepare children for a healthy lifestyle.

Lack of understanding of the youth sports culture, bad food, and an addiction to screens is the three-headed monster attacking our children's health. Despite the excellent data over the past 50 years showing the detrimental effects due to these factors, little has changed. This is not by chance. Powerful advertising and lobbying efforts have kept our children in front of screens and unhealthy foods on our tables, just as they have kept school budgets funding sports, not PE ("Approximately How Much Money," 2010). Schools that have adopted a cultural change in PE (daily, high-energy exercise), as well as getting ultra-processed foods out of the cafeteria, have measured not just improvement in overall student health, but improved performance in the classroom as well. This change should be implemented not just in a few enlightened schools but worldwide, and especially in poorer school districts where other activity options might be limited.

We can solve our health crisis by harnessing something *positive* that is already in our genes. This is an *active* solution that can have a lifelong effect. Negative, passive solutions such as "don't spend so much time on the computer" or "eat more vegetables" are simply not working. Maintaining physical identity before the age of 18 has the best chance of ensuring healthy habits into the future and giving our children the joyful, long life they deserve.

PHYSICAL IDENTITY AND THE PRIMITIVE BRAIN

Children from many Western countries born today will have a shorter lifespan than their parents (Ludwig, 2017). This has never happened before in modern human history. Because homo sapiens have no natural predators and can control their surroundings with remote control, we now completely ignore our hunter-gatherer past. This control has not changed human biology, however, as it has remained fairly static for thousands of years. One of the biggest risk factors for a shortened life is being born in the 21st century. *An 18-year-old today is less healthy than an 18-year-old 200,000 years ago.* Let that sink in for a minute. Despite our terrific doctors, dentists, medicines, baby formulas, antiseptics, and anything else you can think of that has made us "civilized," teenagers today are not as healthy as their hunter-gatherer ancestors. Assuming they made it to 18 (surviving childbirth and the occasional leopard attack), our ancestors' lifestyle of activity and eating a wide variety of foods would put them near the top of the list today for any track coach or military recruiter. So, what happened? In a nutshell, humans did not evolve fast enough to keep pace with Madison Avenue, or more specifically, we could not defeat the scourges of automation, processed foods, and popular video games like *Fortnite.* The three previous revolutions of agriculture, industry, and technology have all been detrimental to our health. We need a revolution that works with Mother Nature and *improves* our health. We need a PE revolution.

As the medical establishment, my colleagues and I must take particular blame. We have been so busy playing whack-a-mole with disease, we failed to notice that there is more to health than building bigger hospitals. So much energy was spent working *against* Mother Nature, we forgot that the vast majority of the time she is working *with* us. She gave us a huge brain that learns to cooperate with other humans. She allowed us to develop big gluteal muscles to run long distances. She installed a great immune system (when we do not poison it with tobacco, sugar, and other toxins). Sometimes health is more primitive, more basic, than we give it credit for.

My goal in this book is to avoid discussing the same things you read and hear on what seems like a daily basis regarding the state of fitness and health in America. What I will emphasize instead is the connection of the health crisis to the limited evolution of our primitive brains and other primitive organ systems. I will also emphasize a human trait that has very much evolved in our brain: identity. The case will be made that holding on to our *physical identity*—that is, holding on to our connection to the outdoors and nature and *motion* as homo sapiens—might be the only solution for a healthy future as a species. Later in this chapter I will point out one striking example of how limiting physical identity and PE could have implications for us as a nation: the state of our military.

THE POWER OF PLAY

Everything we do as humans is informed by our culture and society, which in turn has a huge effect on our identity. But surely there must be some nature in addition to the nurture. Is there some baseline genetic imprint that influences our physical identity? Yes. Despite your university degree, soft bed, and hot running water, you can still see large parts of your "primitive brain" on display daily. One does not need to meet a mountain lion to trigger our ancient fight or flight mechanism. Try driving a car in any city to witness humans in touch with similar primitive instincts! What we have in the 21st century is a combination of primitive and cognitive brain impulses that come into conflict on a daily basis (Greene et al., 2004). We are still guided by primitive brain responses even if we avoid that walk in the woods or driving a car. Our primitive brains dawn each day as the sun rises. These circadian rhythms are hardwired and cannot be displaced by technology, as many people have discovered during northern latitude winters or the hospital night shift (Begemann et al., 1997). Not appreciating the primitive aspect of our brain that shares decisionmaking with the cognitive aspect is a big factor bringing us to the health crisis we have today. But this disconnect with our primitive brain is not our natural state. It gets lost in society's influences. When in our natural state, we move, and when children, we *play.*

certainly not square dancing, but racing around the gym. Like children who play with the box on Christmas morning, moving in our own bodies seemed to be the purest form of fun. We did not want to stand around *learning* how to do something—we wanted to *run*. If we did not run around the gym, we ran around outside at recess, and then we ran around after school. We only went inside with a threat. This was what we did. This was who we were. Unknowingly, we were maintaining our *physical identity*: we played outside—we were in motion.

SOCIETY AND IDENTITY

"When we see anything in any place in one instant of time, we are sure . . . that it is that very thing and not another. . . . And in this consists *identity* . . ."

—John Locke

Developing an identity is a complex undertaking. A combination of intrinsic factors—for instance, gender—but also extrinsic influences—family members, peer groups, and, of course, teachers—come into play (Tsang et al., 2012). Identity is something that is built, not something that just happens. The development of identity can go on to have a positive or negative effect on a child's self-esteem, achievement, social acceptance, and other traits that can last through adulthood (Leahy, 1985). Understanding that a young person is building his or her identity on a daily basis should encourage parents and teachers to conceptualize this development. Ideally, they can influence a student's identity construction for the better on both a personal and societal level (Harter, 1999).

Louis Menand wrestles with societal and other issues of identity in his article about the cultural anthropologist, Margaret Mead (Menand, 2019):

[I]dentity seems to be a concept that lies beyond both culture and biology. Is identity innate, or is it socially constructed? Is it fated, or can it be chosen or performed? Are our identities defined by the existing state of social relations, or do we carry them with us wherever we go? (p. 86)

Perhaps there is no challenge to a child's identity greater than when parents begin to share their complete influence over their daughter or son's life with the local school. In one day in September, their youngster starts being molded by bus drivers, teachers, principals, custodians, and most notably, a class full of peers. This is when things get complicated.

CHILDREN AND IDENTITY

Back in the day, every youngster who played baseball loved Derek Jeter, and for good reason. He was handsome, he was a great teammate, he was modest, and of course, he was the best shortstop of his day. My friend's first grader was no different, though it turns out there was a conflict: We live in New Hampshire. I brought him back a Derek Jeter T-shirt after a trip to Yankee Stadium. He was delighted and proudly pulled it on the next morning and headed for school. Who would have imagined another 6-year-old would take offense and punch poor Sam in the nose, claiming him to be a traitor to the Red Sox? This pugilist was a child with some significant identity as a fan. But what are some of the other identities he is building?

Early in life, children define their identity by a list of characteristics they have been taught about themselves:

- I am a redhead.
- I am from South Philly.
- I am a second grader.
- I am Jewish.
- I am a Red Sox fan!

As if this were not enough, we then ask them to predict their identity as an adult. "What do you want to be when you grow up?" is a question we've all been asked, practically as soon as we can talk. Of course, children will then typically name options they are aware of: firefighter, singer, soccer player, artist, teacher, builder, doctor. Most youngsters, of course, will not end up doing any of these jobs, but some scaffolding for future identity might already be there. Children begin with concrete definitions of identity before they gradually develop a more nuanced, complex, personal, but still culturally influenced understanding. Identity is not rigid, but our concept of self at any one time can play a huge role in what direction our lives take.

One of the first markers of identity that young people have control over is identifying as "athlete" or "nonathlete." It would be the unusual child who at age 6 notes herself to have a passion for math or history. Children, however, know they like to play, since this is what they have been doing for as long as they can remember. A percentage of children start organizing their play: modeling what they see on TV and assimilating the influence of their parents (e.g., keeping a score playing games), leading these children to identify as "athletes," even at an early age.

Athletic identity, as defined by Professor Britton Brewer is "the degree to which an individual identifies with the athlete role . . . the athletic identity construct is discussed within the framework of a multidimensional self-concept" (Brewer et al., 1993). Dr. Brewer goes on to note that "incompetence in a domain of high perceived importance, on the other hand, can profoundly affect one's feelings of self-worth." Incompetence in athletics has the potential to affect feelings of self-worth well into the future (Grove et al., 1997). Studies show that children are not ready for skill games such as baseball until at least the age of 6, and we also know that all 6-year-olds are not at the same physical maturity level (Merkel, 2013). A child who is 6 years and 1 month is significantly less mature than a child who is 6 years and 11 months. In the book *Outliers,* Malcolm Gladwell presents an enlightening discussion of this topic (2009). Researching the sport of ice hockey, he was able to follow the thread of "older" athletes (by months) who kept their playing-time advantage all the way through youth sports to the National Hockey League. Although some have questioned his conclusions, the key here is that children are being categorized (and thus *identified and identifying)* far too early—whether that is being bad at math or good at athletics. Let me remind you: *These are children: They are not good or bad at anything yet!*

Children, like the family dog, are excellent observers. They realize early in life that athletics can have real-world importance in their social status. Many fathers will announce their child's game-winning basket in public and be congratulated by other parents; rarely the case with a good grade on a science test. Which is not to say that all youth and their parents put significant importance on athletics. However, when big sections of newspapers and TV are devoted to sports, and youngsters see numerous people daily wearing the local college or professional team's colors, they get the message. Athletic identity has been shown to be relevant across a lifetime, which is why we must influence this identity as early as possible.

Youngsters are also constantly making comparisons that can impact their identity and sense of self. Am I as smart as the other

students? Are my clothes right? Is my skin color different? Am I shorter than my classmates? But these are assessments being made by the
child. There is a difference when adults are making the comparisons.
Adults prize, discuss, and give great value to athletics—something that
is evident even to young students (see Red Sox fan above). Children
hear parents bragging about how they were "naturals" when they got
in the water, just as they will hear they are "not tough enough" for
hockey. Fewer people worry about what books their 1st-grader is or
isn't reading—they do care how coordinated their child seems on the
ball field. Also, children understand athletics because sports are a form
of play, the one realm in their early lives where they might consider
themselves "experts."

Imagine the girl who watches peers hitting a ball while she herself
has no luck. Putting a child in a competitive situation before they are
ready can cause anxiety and stress, not only diminishing enjoyment
in the short term, but risk eliminating, not just their athletic, but more
importantly, their physical identity, for the long term (Purcell, 2005).
This is why it is dangerous to conflate sports with playing. Not every
child needs to do competitive sports. Every child needs to play.

UNCLE SAM MAY NOT ACTUALLY WANT YOU!

The addition of aggressive PE for every child, every day, is not just
an academic argument relating to school children. Our lack of fitness
could actually become a national security issue. Though this was a
concern throughout the 20th century, the lack of fitness then was
nothing compared to our present generation. We were not talking
about type II diabetes and high blood pressure in teenagers in those
days. Do we dare ask if our present lack of activity and poor food
choices make us vulnerable as a nation? Could our poor physical education be responsible for unprepared armed forces?

These questions have in fact been asked and considered by our military. Major General Allen Batschelet at the Army Recruiting Command
notes that more than 71% of America's youth would not qualify for
the military due to numerous issues, with physical issues, most specifically obesity, as the leading issue (Feeney, 2014). Gregory Poland, MD,
a physician who worked with the government on this topic, supports
this conclusion. Dr. Poland's research found that "one out of three
young adults of military recruitment age in the United States is too

overweight to enlist," going on to say obesity is the "number one cause of ineligibility in the armed services" and that that number was rising on a yearly basis. Major General Batschelet feels such a situation could place our all-volunteer military model at risk.

In terms of obesity, adults are even worse off than children. According to the U.S. Department of Health and Human Services, the number of American adults who are overweight or obese is hovering around *two out of three* (National Institute of Diabetes and Digestive and Kidney Diseases, 2017). Lack of activity, whether in our vocations or avocations, is a major factor. This is incredibly significant since over $147 *billion* in health care costs are associated with obesity (The Healthcare Costs of Obesity). However, you do not need statistics to realize people are out of shape; just look around at the beach or in an airport.

Surgeons especially notice obesity as fatter people make for bigger surgical risks—from infections to blood clots to wearing out their artificial joints faster than they might otherwise. No surgeon wants a complication or bad outcome any more than the patient does. As a result, some surgeons are simply refusing to do certain elective operations such as knee replacements on a patient who is morbidly obese. But at least today's adults probably had years of activity before the technological revolution. Not so with our youngsters.

As appreciated by multiple presidents, and continued with First Lady Michelle Obama, the solutions to these problems are difficult, as so much damage has been done to our present generation. I myself am taking multiple blood pressure tablets daily even though I am not overweight, I exercise regularly, and gave up smoking a long time ago. Growing up, my mother, not exactly a passionate cook, took advantage of many of the "benefits" of the processed and easy-to-prepare foods that gained popularity in the 1950s. I then spent my teen years working at Howard Johnson's and Burger King restaurants. My recovery after summer football practice was to work the drinks station, guzzling Coca Cola (not exactly a "Breakfast of Champions"). Of course, I have made changes to my diet over the years, though perhaps not soon enough for my blood vessels. I suspect many readers are in the same boat.

How does a human organism respond to today's technology revolution? We are asking it to accept inputs it does not understand. Our primitive brains and organs have adapted to all sorts of climate and habitat changes over the millennia, but those are millennia! If you gave me a few thousand years, I would have thought of something really funny and cutting to say when Tommy started kissing my (then) girlfriend at the dance. But I only had seconds, and mumbling "you're a jerk" before storming away was the best I could come up with. My reaction simply did not have enough time to evolve. This is similar to the situation with our bodies. We have added a crazy new set of changes and stresses. The responses to these stresses have led to blood vessel damage in the form of heart disease and stroke, gut issues leading to obesity and bowel disease, and brain deterioration leading to a higher incidence of Alzheimer's, and overall, a shorter lifespan (Alzheimer's Association, 2020; National Cancer Institute, 2015; Shen et al., 2015). These changes are an inflammatory response with damage being done on a consistent and measurable basis, even to a juvenile body. This is why suddenly young people are getting the "Western diseases" of diabetes, high blood pressure, higher levels of depression, ulcers, and other maladies never before seen in youth. Unlike smoking where the cumulative damaging effects manifest after many years and vary from person to person, the anatomic changes to our children's health from a poor diet and inactivity are happening now, and the ravages are appearing far sooner.

I appreciate that there are a host of psychological and sociological factors contributing to obesity, but we simply cannot let this keep us from making changes. Obesity is far more than an aesthetic or social issue—it is a health issue. According to the website for the National Association to Advance Fat Acceptance (NAAFA):

> Fat people are discriminated against in all aspects of daily life, from employment to education to access to public accommodations, and even access to adequate medical care. This discrimination occurs despite evidence that 95 to 98 percent of diets fail over five years and that 65 million Americans are labeled "obese." Our thin-obsessed society firmly believes that fat people are at fault for their size and it is politically correct to stigmatize and ridicule them. (NAAFA, 2016)

As horrible as discrimination might be, obesity should not be thought of only as a social label. It is much more complicated than that. Ultimately though, obesity must be considered a health issue with the myriad diseases that stem from it. One concern not always connected with obesity but seen in high numbers in overweight folks is depression. According to the Centers for Disease Control and

Prevention (CDC), the rate of obesity in those with depression was 10% greater than in those without depression. They go on to note ". . . studies have shown a bidirectional relationship, meaning obesity increases risk of depression and depression increases risk of obesity" (Pratt & Brody, 2015).

We are burdening a child allowed to become obese with a problem that is not only societal, but physical and psychological. I do not want to undervalue the complexity of this topic. I fully appreciate the multiple factors of culture, diet, biology, technology, learned behaviors, societal pressures, school and government policies, and others at play here. That said, we still need to avoid allowing obesity to become the norm, to become an identity. Nothing in human evolution can be considered inherent after only 50 years or two generations, basically the length of the obesity crisis.

It might be too late for us older folks and perhaps even today's teenagers to be healthy. This generation may indeed be beyond repair. This does not have to be the case for our youngest students and the next generation. For much of my life, I have had great timing. For our children, the time for them to get healthy is fading each day they are not in motion, each day they spend indoors. We have the knowledge, we have the technology, we have the infrastructure, we have the means, and we have the personnel to make necessary changes so that the *next* generation does not have to suffer the same fate, or worse. What we need now is the will and energy to start the next revolution: the health revolution, the PE revolution. Culture, similar to identity, is not immutable. Yes, everything in our lives and brains are affected on some level by the way of life around us. A culture, however, can change as circumstances change, and our world in the 21st century is not the same one we left after the Y2K party. In short, most of us are "average," and thus we need a social system that works for the majority of those students not at the top end of the bell curve.

CHAPTER 2

The Rise and Fall of Physical Education

EVIDENCE-BASED PHYSICAL EDUCATION: WHY REBRANDING IS NEEDED

The world changed. This change has brought us to a crisis point regarding children's health, and our stubbornness as a society is keeping us from addressing it. Like Janus, we are forever looking forward and back. On one level, we long for the "good old days," yet no one would wish to go back 100 or even 50 years to an unreliable electric grid, summers without air conditioning, or, perhaps the worst cut of all, life without the Internet (then again . . .). Perhaps the one thing many of us would like to go back to are lives of more outdoor play and activity. But, as Janus's Greek friend Pandora would attest, we cannot pick and choose the things we want to change and the things we do not. As we discussed, one of the brain functions humans have developed is *flexibility*. It is just this flexibility that has allowed us to adapt, with varied success, to our lives today (except for Great Aunt Delia—she will never change!).

My own field of medicine was stuck for *centuries* without progress. Religious beliefs, political wrangling, laws against dissection, and, perhaps most pointedly, fear, kept doctors fixated on the "four humors," with bleeding a common treatment for many ailments. This is not to say in medicine today we have completely given ourselves to progress, as there is a tendency to cling to methods we have learned from our elders, just as they did from theirs. Luckily, however, there is now enough impetus in the field of medicine to assure change and steady progress moving forward. It is the rare doctor who does not keep up with the published literature (especially knowing in the age of Google that if he or she does not, their patients will!). Most specialty boards (specialties meaning fields such as obstetrics, internal medicine, dermatology, etc.)

require physicians to pass some type of test every 10 years, thus ensuring they keep abreast of an ever-expanding bank of knowledge. In my own case of orthopedics and sports medicine, every decade I can either answer a live panel of questioners or sit for a written exam. Neither is easy, but once successfully completed, you can proudly call yourself "board certified" by your academy.

As another prod encouraging physicians to use science, not just training, to inform their treatment choices, the use of evidence-based medicine (EBM) is now emphasized in every specialty (Masic et al., 2008). That is not to say that previous knowledge is discarded. EBM combines both the clinical experience and the best available research for making decisions regarding patient care. EBM insists that the research used for medical decisionmaking be of high quality, necessitating accurate data collection, large samples when available, and strict statistical methods. With English being the almost universal language of medicine, and the Internet connecting us to EBM research around the globe, doctors have access to an incredible wealth of knowledge, not just that being published in the United States.

In theory, the use of EBM should ensure consistency in care across a medical specialty. "Best practices" is a term to connote a similar concept to "evidence-based." Best practices makes it no longer acceptable to do something "because that's the way I have always done it" or because it was the way one of your professors did it. This is not to say that all physicians pay attention to EBM recommendations. My own study on opioid narcotic prescriptions after knee surgery had been largely ignored until recently, when opioid abuse became national news (O'Neill & Thomas, 2014).

When it comes to children's health, we are guilty as a society of ignoring the evidence-based knowledge in the face of a crisis. We know the statistics from America and around the world. Despite finally recognizing this problem, no significant progress to alter this horror is being made. As discussed, obesity is just one easy measure to assess general health. It is often associated with high blood pressure, diabetes, high cholesterol, psychological issues, lowered immunities, and a host of other afflictions. In the last chapter I presented the case for physical identity as inherent to our being. *It is my contention that the maintenance of our physical identity is vital for escaping this web of obesity and poor health trapping our youth.* A school's physical education (PE) program should be a key component to continue and develop physical identity, but the PE system is stuck in the past.

Here are some of the questions we will be examining as we make the case for a change in our PE system to address the health crisis:

- What is the history of PE in America that brought us to our present state?
- How has PE in our public schools changed in the past century?
- What effect are organized sports having on PE in our schools?
- Where are the data showing the effectiveness of our PE programs in both health and academic performance?
- How is evidenced-based learning being utilized in the average PE class?
- Are we able to create a change in the PE culture and delivery with present school budgets?
- Can we "rebrand" PE with a new identity to connote what it really should be representing?

Before tackling these and other admittedly tough questions, let me first make the case for why we need a revolution: *A child born today will be able to live his or her entire life without doing anything physical*. Nothing. Janus does not have to look back far to see this change. Let us go back just 50 years to compare youth activity then with youth activity today.

WHAT WE DO NOT DO IN OUR DAILY LIVES (BABY BOOMERS TAKE NOTE!)

- Get up to answer the phone.
- Crank down a car window.
- Shift a manual transmission.
- Wash and dry the dishes.
- Go to the mailbox for the newspaper and letters.
- Manually change the TV channel.
- Walk into a shop to make a purchase.
- Go to a restaurant where you actually get out of the car.

We could play this game for quite a while. For the compulsives out there, you would be able to collect a list of well over 30 items in less than 5 minutes. (P.S. Farmers are not allowed to play!) Except in certain states, basically the only thing we do now that was histori- cally done for us is to pump our own gas. The importance of this list is that each of these seemingly minor movements have a calorie count attached, and these calories add up at the end of the day. This is not a reflection of any increased laziness, but simply advances in technology ("modern conveniences") eliminating many of the manual tasks that forced us to use energy without a conscious effort.

If we just look at these everyday activities (forgetting for now annual activities such as storm windows, stacking wood, putting in the garden, etc.), *a person today will burn roughly 200 fewer calories a day than someone 50 years ago!* Over the course of a year, this could add up to some 20 pounds of weight. Again, these are calories not being burned due to new efficiencies introduced in the past 50 years—changing what the medical community calls "activities of daily living," or the basic tasks of everyday life. In the case of our children, we are not asking them to adjust for burning fewer calories with a longer and more aggressive PE class or recess—just the opposite. Not only has the overall time for PE shrunk, but how much of that limited time the students *actually spend moving* is less and less.

This use of technology and lack of motion can have other health implications besides obesity. It can also lead to what Professor Avery Faigenbaum calls "pediatric dynapenia" (a "poverty of strength") (Faigenbaum & Macdonald, 2017). Dr. Faigenbaum puts dynapenia on one arm of the "pediatric inactivity triad," with exercises deficit disorder (less than 60 minutes daily) and physical illiteracy (lack of competence and confidence in movements) on the other two arms (Faigenbaum et al., 2018). Thus a child without obesity may appear "healthy" when only looking at the body mass index (BMI) statistics, but their lack of motion and muscle mass can still lead to poor health. And now it becomes a disease loop. Having obesity or pediatric inactivity leads a child to seek *less* physical activity, which leads to more childhood disease, which leads to greater obesity and inactivity. All this to say, it is time to stop thinking we Americans are the tough pioneer, rugged outdoorsman, streetwise, grizzled Yankee types with a Puritan work ethic. America leads the world in pediatric obesity and pediatric inactivity; we're not nearly as tough as we think!

WHAT CHILDREN DO NOT DO AFTER SCHOOL

The answer to this is seemingly easy: *They do not go out and play.* But wait! Once again, as with most of these topics, it is actually a bit more complicated.

A child growing up 50 years ago quickly conquered his or her immediate indoor environment, and after that, anything of real interest was one place: *outside*. Back in the day (I put in that phrase to get an eye roll from anyone under the age of 40) we wanted to be outside and find adventures like in the stories we were reading of Nancy Drew, *Call of the Wild*, and the Hardy Boys. Add the plethora of biographies about heroes like Jesse Owens, Sacagawea, Amelia Earhart, and others, and there was never a reason to be indoors—fame, fortune, and adventure lay beyond the front door and down the road—never in a bedroom or anywhere near your parents! Fifty years ago in America, at best there were three uninteresting TV channels, annoying siblings (it was the baby boom), and the possibility of being asked to do chores. The goal, once a certain level of independence was reached, was to get out into the larger world. For this author, outdoors meant touch-football games in the fall, basketball once the ground was hard enough to bounce the ball, a short hockey season when the ponds froze, and myriad baseball games of limitless imagination depending on how many bodies were available. (This included the famed three-person game known to be played only in the backyard at 64 East 16th Street, "Grounder to Short.") Other times, there were forts to be built, hikes to be conquered, bikes to ride, and fierce battles to be fought with army soldiers, as World War II was still fresh in everyone's consciousness. As an added bonus—children outside being busy have little time or interest in eating—they are too busy playing. Such behavior can be seen in most dogs. Dogs are interested in eating from a bowl at home only when not in the woods hunting for real food!

Such is not the case today, but why? Again, the answer is complicated. With apologies to those sociologists who have made this their lifelong research, I will try to summarize the problem in a few pages. We will attempt to get our arms around what is to my mind a two-part problem. One is technological and the other is cultural. The technological problem is the most extraordinary topic of modern times: the rise of the computer.

Their World Is Flat

First, let me make a confession to my younger readers (there might be one or two). I have no idea of how addicting video games, Twitter, Snapchat, Hulu, Instagram, and so on, truly are. That said, I suspect by the time this book is published, at least one of these will be yesterday's news. Time in front of any two-dimensional entertainment platform is one of the main antagonists in this health drama. Most of us over a certain age just do not know why young people are obsessed with these venues because they were simply not part of our lives. This is changing though, as few among us abstain from at least some daily computer time (Anderson & Perrin, 2017). Although this might be lamentable on many levels for older folks, when involving young-sters, the addiction to screens has cost them their health. According to government data, children now spend more than *7 1/2 hours a day* in front of a screen (e.g., TVs, video games, computers, smartphones) (Anderson, 2018). Let me remind the reader—there are 24 hours in a day, and they still need to eat and sleep! Regarding the latter, the American Academy of Pediatrics (AAP) recommendation for sleep time is 9–12 hours for children 6–12 years old, and 8–10 hours for teens (American Academy of Pediatrics Supports Childhood Sleep Guidelines, 2016).

Staying with my pediatric colleagues, let's look at some data from an AAP policy statement from 2016, "Media Use in School-Aged Children and Adolescents," regarding screen time (Council on Communications and Media). To summarize:

- Three quarters of teenagers own a smartphone.
- One quarter of teens consider themselves *"constantly connected"* to the Internet.
- Four fifths of households have a video game device.
- The odds of being overweight are almost five times greater for adolescents who watch more than 5 hours of TV per day, compared to those watching 0 to 2 hours, thus the AAP recommends *2 hours or less of sedentary screen time daily.* Furthermore, screen time and psychological well-being are directly related. The more screen time, the more mental health issues (Boers, 2019).

Game play is ubiquitous across all teens. Nearly one third of high school students play video or computer games for 3 or more hours on an average school day. Sadly, boys, who seem to be falling behind more and more academically, play games more often and for longer periods of time than the girls.

We could go on with such statistics, and, depending on what new research you look at, you can become more and more horrified.

Screen time, combined with fast food, make two incredibly worthy foes that cannot be contained without a cultural revolution. (P.S. They will never be "defeated.")

MOTHER NATURE TO THE RESCUE

Mother Nature can compete with this screen siren because *in our primitive brain there is the need to get outside.* Although not on the level of wild animals, we are not so far removed. We literally crave nature, and our brains respond to it in a powerful way (Williams, 2017). Edmund O. Wilson called this *biophilia,* the "urge to affiliate with other forms of life" (2003). As good as video games get, they cannot approach the feedback our brains receive from nature. An analogy one can consider is all the talk about robots and artificial intelligence taking over human tasks. Trust me, just the human *hand* is a structure that will never be replicated by robots to even 50% of what it actually does. The movement, dexterity, solace, protection, identification, and a host of other jobs of the hand are many millennia from being replicated by a robot. Feeling nature with your hands in addition to your eyes, your ears, and your nose stimulates the primitive brain. Video games try to replicate natural outdoor stimuli, but by definition will always fall short (and "outside" can be as simple as a city park). A positive change I have seen in my lifetime are American communities appreciating the importance of green spaces and waterfront areas. We must, as a society, present our children with these healthy alternatives. We do not have to beat young people over the head with this. Just allow their brains, hands, and feet (take off those shoes!) to engage, and Mother Nature will do the rest. Although they might not always make healthy choices, they will more often when they know what is outside and how good they feel connecting with it. Nobody ever regrets a walk on the beach.

THEY DON'T HAVE TIME, AND IT'S DANGEROUS

After technology, the second major impediment to not playing outside is cultural, and, I contend, something we can more easily affect. This is actually a topic of research in essentially all postindustrial countries, including the United States, the Netherlands, Sweden, Portugal, Ireland, the United Kingdom, and others. These studies are in agreement that children playing outside is a positive and to be encouraged (Ginsberg, 2007; Prince et al., 2013). Play has been linked to increased brain function, improved coordination, and teaching cooperation and deci- sionmaking, yet it is disappearing from our children's lives. But why the disconnect? Most parents want their children to play outside sim- ply because *they* played outside in their own youth and remember the joy it brought. Children's brains will imprint a visit to a museum or a day body surfing far stronger than another hour in front of a screen. Despite the research and parents universally wanting their children to play more outside, there are multiple roadblocks to this happening.

In many cases, the roadblock to outdoor play is the child's sched- ule. A huge percentage are simply too busy with sports, ballet, and other activities organized by their parents. I have done my own strictly nonscientific survey over the years, asking multiple relatives, friends, and patients about their children's packed calendar. Try this survey yourself in your own social circle. I suspect the answers will be similar:

- "I want to keep them busy and out of trouble."
- "Otherwise, there is nothing for them to do." (This answer gives me PTSD. I learned early in life never to use the word "bored" around my father.)
- "It's part of my own social life—I like watching them play." (a member of President Kennedy's "nation of spectators?")
- "I remember how I behaved when I was their age, and don't want them acting the same." (No, I usually do not follow up on this answer.)
- "If I don't organize something, all they will do is watch TV and play video games."
- "Otherwise they will bug me."
- "They might get eaten by a bear." (The last time someone was killed by a bear in New Hampshire was the 18th century—and I suspect even that was "wilderness legend.")
- "There are just too many crazies running around."

But these children are actually the lucky ones—their parents mean well and they are given options for after-school activities. Too many of our young people are not offered such opportunities, and thus by design are spending afternoons confined to their homes as opposed to roaming the outdoors as children—urban, suburban, and rural—did in my generation. When I ask this subgroup of parents the reason for such confinement, the answer is always the same: fear. Fear is expressed in numerous studies, particularly from poor socioeconomic areas. Public housing, parental mental health diagnoses, perception of neighborhood safety (how much crime we *think* is being committed), and loss of public trust were all factors for keeping children indoors (Aarts et al., 2012). Facility accessibility was not as strong a reason as one might guess, though making play areas safer and more interesting is always a plus and something communities should continue to explore (Kalish et al., 2010; Kimbro & Schachter, 2011). Although fear of bear attacks may well be overblown, the safety concerns of low-income families in predominantly urban and rural areas provide all the more reason to build strong, innovative PE programs in our schools that get students outside whenever possible.

An urban parent responds:

We don't give him a ton of leisure time, we don't provide windows of time for independent play, we don't give him many opportunities to become bored—and then learn how to entertain himself. Certainly not in the outdoors! And we (I) do feel a little guilty about this, because I grew up in the middle of the woods with nothing to do, ever, and no one to do anything with, and I learned how to find ways to keep myself busy, and I feel like I'm better for it. But if we don't sign up for these sports and clinics and classes, then we end up getting stuck inside with an increasingly impatient, under-stimulated child. Organized activities make things really easy, and our kid loves seeing his friends and knowing he's going to play with them at specific times every weekend.

One nice thing about urban playgrounds is that kids play in them! All kinds of kids. The playgrounds in the city are beautifully demographic. You get this great melting pot of kids from different backgrounds or socioeconomic groups playing together—especially if someone has a ball.

WHAT WE DO NOT DO FOR WORK

Might there still be hope after high school to get our human organisms fit and healthy with years of hard work? Well, yes, though such is not often the case.

It is the rare occupation in the United States that has not been made easier (and hopefully at the same time, safer) by our oft-dreaded technology. In addition to work in general getting less physical, according to the Pew Research Center, job growth is distinctly not trending toward calorie-burning occupations such as farming and manufacturing (DeSilver, 2017). New job growth is much stronger in education, health care, and professional services. Although these can be tiring, they are not the grueling, heavy, "back-breaking" type of work we associate with big muscles and strong bones.

So there we have it: A baby born in essentially any postindustrial society starts out as any other active animal—in motion and exploring the world. When they get to school though, the motion anchor is dropped. Here, activity involves perhaps two gym classes a week (if they are lucky), a short recess, and home to an afternoon playing video games and texting friends. For the privileged child, this will be supplemented by dance class, karate, youth sports, or some other activity depending on location, parental interest, time, and money. After the age of 13 only about 30% of children who participate in youth sports will go on to play organized school sports (Miner, 2019; SHAPE America Society of Health and Physical Educators, n.d.). Many of these youngsters will have been turned off by the commitment, competition, fear of failure, and expense of sports and choose to participate in other "activities," with the biggest option being the video screen. The vast majority of high school graduates will then find a job that in all likelihood does not entail heavy labor. Later, they will be treated for diabetes, osteoporosis, and a host of other maladies due to this lack of movement. But the heavily scheduled children mentioned earlier, surely they must come out fine? Maybe we just need to increase that percentage to get us out of this crisis?

If only it were that easy.

THE ADULTING OF YOUTH PLAY

You will start to notice a theme that will be pervasive as we discuss the activity evolution of our youngsters. At each stage of youth development in the past century, money and adults take on a larger role, and actual "play" a lesser role. From the time adults took over interscholastic competitions, to the loss of community club teams, to the rise of national youth sports organizations, to the building of enormous public school stadia, to the race for college scholarships, to the selling of TV rights for high school games—*adults and money*—not health and fun, has worked itself front and center.

The topic of play has been broached in multiple forms already, starting quite literally at the beginning, comparing human play to that of other species. I argued that play was the definition of *natural*, as even octopi have been observed to participate. This primitive play instinct, however, has not discouraged some American entrepreneurs from jostling to be on the tip of the spear of our youth sports-industrial complex. For example, in one community in Michigan, if you feel your baby is "play challenged," you can enroll the infant in a class to teach him or her "physical literacy" (this is not a joke, and yes, you will need your credit card). There is a story someone once told about the great Laurence Olivier. When a younger actor in the movie was describing the trials of self-deprivation he put himself through to prepare for his role, Sir Laurence is said to have replied, "My boy, wouldn't it be easier just to *act*?" Likewise, rather than paying someone to teach your baby physical literacy, wouldn't it be easier just to *play* with her? This idea of a baby needing physical literacy might represent the pinnacle of the "adulting" of play. I might suggest the parents save their money and learn from the play expert there in the crib, but perhaps that is a different book!

This monetization of a baby's natural state is perhaps the inevitable outcome of our shift away from play and toward organized sports. Previously, we emphasized that "play" (sometimes called "free play") should be distinguished from sports, which at best would be labeled "organized play." For the purpose of this discussion, we will define organized youth sports as a physical activity with a set of rules governed and supervised by adults, involving uniforms, competitions, and the goal of winning. So next on our list regarding the adulting of play is just that: *organized sports*. Though here's the rub: Not every child participates. This journey from play to organized sports, and the parallel journey from public school PE to organized sports, has excluded a big chunk of the population (Swanson, 2017). *This evolution of organized sports over the past 50 years is now to the point where it is one of the major factors hindering the health of our children, both physically and psychologically.*

How did sports, thought to be an incredibly positive thing, become a hindrance to children's health? The main factor is that once a child ceases to participate in sports they lose their identity as an athlete. And loss of identity as an athlete in the 21st century almost always means loss of *physical identity as an active human being.* This is where the trouble really begins.

What is the opposite of an athlete? A nonathlete. With no organized sports to participate in, all too often there exists in that young person's life no activity and thus no motion, leading to the pediatric inactivity triad and often obesity. "Nonathletes" do not play outside after school. They do not ride bikes, hike, ski, swim, or simply explore the natural world. Nonathletes in today's world turn on the computer (the new "play"). *Our job is to not allow children to lose their physical identity and commit themselves to a life in front of a screen.* So before moving forward, let's look at the history that paved the way for Apple and Xbox to take over play; why youngsters self-segregate into athlete and nonathlete due to the emphasis on competitive sports; and the tender subject of how the "varsity" sports model might not be appropriate for most high schools.

A SYSTEM PUT IN PLACE FOR A VERY DIFFERENT TIME

Before going any further, let me acknowledge that I am not any more a historian than I am a sociologist, and this is not meant to be a complete dossier of the U.S. educational and school athletic systems' past. I will attempt, however, with broad strokes, to show where we have been and where we are now regarding our nonprofessional organized sports and PE. There are some wonderful scholarly works on this subject that are referenced throughout.

At the turn of the last century, millions of immigrants were flowing into the ports of New York, Boston, Philadelphia, New Orleans, San Francisco, and dozens of other coastal cities. From there, many would catch trains to Pittsburgh, Chicago, and beyond. Most were guaranteed employment at growing manufacturing centers, while some were lucky enough to purchase and work their own land. Many of these folks were truly the "wretched refuse" from other countries, which often meant farmers and other unskilled laborers looking for a better life in America (Immigration in the Early 1900s, n.d.). My own grandfather was one of these people. With no work in Ireland, and politically closed out of a chance of owning property, he came through Boston and quickly volunteered to "fight the Kaiser," hoping to gain U.S. citizenship.

As the slums of our cities teemed with children lacking farm chores or other tasks to perform, they quickly became a neighborhood nuisance (Pruter, 2013). The drive for compulsory public education, having started in the mid-1800s, took on new urgency with this spike in population. Now though, educators had an ally in industry. The post–Industrial Revolution economy was in high gear, and the expanding need for educated blue- and white-collar workers was pronounced. It was also near the end of the 1800s that the number of public school students exceeded those at private schools (Krug, 1969). One of my favorite cartoons is a drawing of two chemists looking at a blackboard covered with formulas. In the middle of this is written, "now a miracle happens." Regarding compulsory education, the "miracle" was multiple factors and common interests, including (in no particular order):

- A tenfold increase in the number of students from 1890 to 1920 (Krug, 1969).
- The Rockefellers, Morgans, Carnegies, and other industrial leaders needing loyal and better educated workers (Library of Congress, n.d.).
- The rise of education as a bureaucracy and profession, with dedicated schools directed by education "experts" such as John Dewey ("John Dewey," 2020).
- Groups like the Ku Klux Klan's fear of the influence of parochial schools (Slawson, 2005).
- An interest from politicians to "Americanize" the disparate immigrants with an education that taught more than just "the three Rs" but also emphasized core values to help teach cooperation and loyalty (Krug, 1969).

Once the decision was made that children should be educated, other aspects of school, including free play and PE, as well as their first cousin, sports, were introduced as part of the curriculum. A significant influence for some type of recreation were founders of the "playground movement" who felt that

> recreation not only benefited the individual but also transformed a nation of alien immigrants, or downtrodden, unhealthy factory workers, into a cohesive, healthy, population of citizens working for the common good and ready to defend their country. (Anderson, 2006)

(As discussed in Chapter 1, the health of our potential fighting force seems recently to have taken a backseat to other concerns.)

At the start of the 1900s, there were still many local community club teams that were actually working in cooperation with the growing school team leagues. These were funded by multiple organizations and active even in poor communities (Riess, 2011). When the Great Depression hit, however, many of these local teams disbanded for lack of funds and never returned. After this, the groups that did survive strengthened, such as the YMCA, Little League Baseball, and Pop Warner Football, though in these new iterations they tended to favor children of means (Merkel, 2013).

PHYSICAL EDUCATION AND INTERSCHOLASTIC SPORTS

A great resource for this topic is Robert Pruter's book *The Rise of High School Sports and Search for Control 1880–1930* (Pruter, 2013). In the preface, Mr. Pruter states,

> Through more than a century of our history, high school sports have engaged variously our educators, our medical and psychological experts, our politicians, our military leaders, and our families who have debated their role, their moral worth, their value, their very existence.

Let's look a bit closer at public school sports history here in America as we consider this long-standing debate.

We can trace the influences of our playground movement and public school sports system back to the private school system here in the United States, which in turn has its roots in English boarding schools (Pruter, 2013). Similar to our own education evolution, the English system was driven by the economy. Increased wealth in post–Industrial Revolution England allowed more people to send their children to private schools. The connection between the physical, mental, and, in the case of many of these religious-based schools, spiritual, was being recognized (think the original *Goodbye, Mr. Chips*). The concept of connecting a strong spirit and strong body was coined "muscular Christianity." Sports that had started out as free play periods soon came under the influence of student leaders. In addition to building muscle, having the boys (and we are essentially only talking about boys in the English system) burn energy on the playing fields was felt to be good for the students and those trying to teach them, helping presumably eliminate the risk of vice and mischief

(Pruter, 2013). When this program and attitude was adopted here in the United States, the physicality of American football was thought to be especially useful for keeping exuberant boys in line. We will revisit this concept of not just muscular Christianity, but the exclusion of women in aggressive sports when we examine the program at La Sierra High School. Although this gender exclusion has improved with the passage of Title IX in 1972, it still haunts our school sports.

The first outdoor interscholastic sports competitions in America took place between elite private New England schools in the 1850s, just before the Civil War. The building of gymnasiums started to flourish in response to the cold northeast winters, and they appeared on multiple private school campuses by 1900 (Pruter, 2013). Perhaps not surprisingly, given his location near many of these private schools, James Naismith, in 1891, invented one of the more popular indoor sports: basketball. It was the outdoor sports, however, that led the competitive way as the century turned, including baseball, football, and track and field. The games started, especially regarding baseball, with high school students playing against all comers, including community club teams and college freshman teams. Thus we have a history in America of amateur teams representing a locale well before the teams were officially representing the district schools. *This will be important later as we look at options for organized sports today.* The early track meets were referred to as "field days," the same title given to races when I was a boy at Silas Wood Elementary School in the 1960s. Tennis and winter sports were soon added to the interscholastic schedule. After the turn of the century, the standard "calisthenics" and German "gymnasium" with pommel horses, high bars, and other still-familiar equipment was emphasized less, as recreation and fitness pivoted toward competitions (Riess, 1995). *This pivot proves vitally important as it indicates an easing away from the concept of exercise as a health and personal improvement tool toward exercise as team contests.*

The early public school teams, similar to those in the private schools, were run and organized predominantly by the students (Pruter, 2013). Although there was some grumbling from the occasional teacher or administrator regarding the mixing of sport and scholarship, like the compromises from their private school contemporaries, it was hoped that such athletic contests would help produce "virtuous" *men* and "Christians committed to health and manliness" (Pruter, 2013). In the case of immigrants, it was hoped sports would help assimilate them into American society.

In 1903, leaders of the playground movement, along with Dr. Luther Halsey Gulick, helped establish the New York City Public School Athletic League for Boys (PSAL) (Pruter, 2013). To its credit, the PSAL at its inception was not just about interscholastic sports, but participation. The rules required 80% of all students to participate, with winning decided by a class average rather than an individual performance (Pruter, 2013). Also in keeping with the concept of participation for all, football was not part of the PSAL in the early stages. The violence of football was already being debated, and there was a belief it was geared toward elite athletes, as opposed to the average student. This early PSAL system would certainly be in line with my concept of continuing physical identity, as it is a much more inclusive and egalitarian scheme than that seen in school sports today.

Parallel with the move toward compulsory schooling, the turn of the 20th century also saw the formalization of physical education (PE) teaching. Influential figures such as Dr. Dudley A. Sargent became nationally prominent, and the PE profession was taking notice of organized sports (Pruter, 2013). Some in this relatively new profession shared previous educators' concerns that such competitive sporting activities might be detrimental to the Christian morals they felt important. As a result, they sought more of a voice in school sports, which at the time were still predominantly student run. Along the way, interscholastic sports leagues became more formalized and student control was tested (Riess, 1995). The concept of sportsmanship was given lip service, but with no clear guidance regarding what this meant or what form it should take. What was taking shape as an offshoot of the athletic contests at this time were psychological constructs that claimed benefits from competition, such as notions of "school spirit" and "loyalty." Along with these concepts came a perhaps more primitive brain response: the importance of "winning" and even possibly doing "unChristian" things to make this come about.

The trend paralleling the private schools continued in the 1920s, as public schools built indoor athletic facilities that often became the center of community life (Pruter, 2013). Although at first the education building boom took place in urban areas, by the 1920s smaller towns were also erecting schools with attached sports facilities. By this time, athletics had been institutionalized virtually everywhere in America. Perhaps not surprisingly, adults became more involved in school sports as the level of sophistication and complexity of these competitions increased, with adults proving useful to secure the use of facilities, sponsorships, officiating, and other logistics. Thus, while the community leaders and parents slowly lost control over the majority of their children's *scholastic* development to professional educators, they did maintain significant control of interscholastic athletics. By 1940, 50% of students were finishing a high school degree and competitive school sports were part of the American culture.

Organized youth sports at all levels, from schools to national organizations to local church and community leagues, exploded after World War II with the growth of the suburbs. This surely was the second biggest influence on the growth of sports since the population explosion due to immigration 50 years earlier. What could be a more perfect breeding ground for sports than a wealthy postwar economy, a generation looking for escape and leisure from years of war, green playing fields, and a baby boom? This historic change continues today as the majority of organized sports participants are boys and girls from the suburbs, who today are playing in generally equal numbers (Swanson, 2017). Suburban gender equality is the good news. The bad news is that children from rural and urban areas, particularly girls of color, participate in far fewer numbers. The other bad news is that the wealthier children continue to have unequal representation on these sports teams. Aside from the issues of local availability and parental involvement, not every child is able to participate in organized sports due to expense, making PE even more vital for most children. As was stated by Eric Jensen, author of *Enriching the Brain* (2008), another book documenting the link between PE and academic performance:

> The upper echelon in our society will have more access to sports, and the lower income kids will get less and less physical activity. . . . This trend keeps poverty-stricken kids where they are . . . it's not getting better; it's getting worse in our nation.

Some early physical educators saw the nature of competitive sports favoring superior athletes and moving away from the more participatory models such as that of the PSAL. With this conflict between ideologies, the battle for control of school sports took on new energy. The PE community marched under the banner of making athletics part of physical *education*, while many in the community saw athletics as a vehicle for civic pride, Americanization, and career advancement. In other words, school sports were taking on a role distinctly not connected to classroom learning. Although one aspect of

the adult takeover of school sports was purportedly to eliminate un-
toward shenanigans thought to be taking place during competitions,
youth sports were becoming a burgeoning industry with money to
be made (Jensen, 2008). PE teachers were able to hold control of elementary school's limited interscholastic sports schedule; however, at
the high school level, it was and remains a different setup. Sports in
high schools today are controlled by athletic directors and coaches
who may or may not also be teachers (see Chapter 4). If these high
school coaches do not field teams that are successful, their jobs are
often at risk due to community pressures, not pressures from within
the school. Thus interscholastic competitions became, and remain, a
big part of the high school experience with no significant connection
to PE. The financial setup has also remained consistent over the past
50 years. In the primary grades there is a limited schedule and budget
for sports, and they are controlled most often by educators. Parents
pay for the bulk of elementary-age competition through youth sport
organizations. At the high school level, public schools become the pre-
dominant organizer of competitive sports. Here the schedule and budget skyrocket, and the much larger tab is incurred by every taxpayer
in the community.

IN SUPPORT OF ORGANIZED SPORTS:
MAKING IT FUN FOR ALL PARTICIPANTS

Sports as a National Identity

We started this book discussing identity, acknowledging it is not always easy to quantify. As we noted with our baseball fan, identity can
be established on multiple levels, often geographical. Our founding
fathers played a huge part in establishing a *national* identity. Part of this
national identity is having pride in our relatively short history, which
we celebrate with holidays like Martin Luther King Day, President's
Day, and Memorial Day. (My apologies to the Native American readers whose history on this land is measured over millennia, not a few
centuries.) I also appreciate that dominance in organized athletics
such as the summer Olympics is part of that national identity. This aspect of our identity, however, seems to be working against us as there
is an inertia to not make important changes in our system of athletics
even though it might be affecting the nation's overall health. We have

a public school system that develops and rewards the superior athlete, but leaves the majority of students and their physical needs behind. Historically, one of America's identities was that of a forward-thinking country that often represented cultural and political progress to much of the world. It is time to be that country again.

The rebranded public school PE I propose does not rely on sports but on high-energy physical exercise everyday, for every child, to maintain physical identity and graduate healthy young adults. I appreciate this might be a challenge to our national identity, but to my mind offers our best, most economical, and actually *easiest* way to lower the obesity rate, raise academic performance, and increase life expectancy. In an ideal world, organized sports are going to be in addition to a child's active, daily, outdoor life, of which PE is a part when school is in session. Intact physical identity will stimulate all students—those who participate in organized sports and the majority who do not—to seek outdoor activities and make better life choices, including healthier food choices, as they grow. One of the keys to this—and remember we are competing with Silicon Valley—is to access that primitive play gene.

We have all spent time watching youth sports. When the children are very young, it is all about the motion. Launching straight down the ski hill, following the soccer ball like a pack of wolves, trying to score a basket from midcourt when they can barely throw the ball 10 feet, not realizing they have scored a touchdown—this innocence is the best of youth sports. It is pure fun. There is no real score (at least not for the players!), no expectations, and bruises are quickly forgotten with an orange wedge.

These early days are quickly overtaken by obsessed adults (more so than the participants), uniforms, score keeping, and the "better athletes" playing while the others sit on the bench. The literature is clear about what makes for a bad sports experience in the majority of cases: *parents and coaches* (Merkel, 2013). I suspect this does not come as a surprise to anyone who has spent time on a sideline of any sport, for any age group. How did we go from the attitude of fresh air, participation, and *playing*, to the idea that the only thing that matters is "winning?" This is at best a complicated devolution that could be a book unto itself. Certainly, some aspects of the obsession with winning can be traced to the roots of our athletic system, to associating morality with physical dominance, to the culture of America changing with its ranking as a world power, to associating victory on the athletic field with "superiority" and success in life, and to other aspects of sport that have become a national identity. I would ask the readers to add other possibilities to this list regarding this brutally complex but important subject, as I feel it is part of why we are stalled as a culture from moving forward.

The Importance of Good Coaching

Most youth coaches have *experience* with the sport they are coaching. Only a minority have *expertise* or education in this endeavor, and thus they will often approach the job by modeling behavior of other coaches they have seen—professional and Division I college coaches. Now think of our average 6-year-old. This child is interested in playing, not winning. Young (and old!) people want to have fun. They want to engage with the other children, to laugh and be silly. They want to use their primitive brain skills of cooperation and flexibility. They want to get an ice cream cone after the game. Pushing them to win, to put themselves in physical danger they are not ready for, to stand for long periods of time, or worse, to sit for long periods of time (and for youngsters, *seconds* can be long) are the surest ways to get children to lose interest. This has also been shown to create anxiety in children—precisely the opposite of what we want them to experience. In regard to playing time, children know who among them are the better athletes on the team. This does not have to be reinforced by coaches letting those children play more often. Coaches who think they are working with the Celtics or Cowboys or ManU are going to push many players straight to the couch—and this is even more damaging when coaching girls. Coaches can create a negative atmosphere by doting on favorites, emphasizing winning, and demonstrating poor teaching skills. Now consider an option to organized sports: The child could be dominating in his or her own video game with nonstop action!

I spent significant time caring for the women's U.S. Alpine Ski Team and have been the team doctor on the sidelines for many women's competitions, at all levels. Girls and women are processing life differently than boys, and this extends to the athletic field. Any good coach— male or female—knows that unless you appreciate this, things will not go well. Some of my own research supported these gender differences (O'Neill, 2008; O'Neill & Marsden, 2017). A good coach must consider many variables to ensure all players are having a positive experience.

That's the coaches. I will not belabor the point regarding the other adult in the equation often making life difficult for the youth athlete: that of the "little league parent." We have all seen them—and heard them! Even though I have studied psychology, I will never be able to understand why anyone would allow themselves to be that stereotypical parent. There is simply no excuse for being rude to an umpire or referee (who are often volunteering their time), or a player or parent from the opposing team (or your own team!). Such behavior cannot be confused with caring. Adults acting like petulant children on the sideline might be the quickest way to turn youngsters off from sports—or, for that matter, from other activities with their parents. We must use every tool in the box to regain our children's health. Having a bad organized sports experience is like having a bad PE experience—it drives them to the most unhealthy place in the world: the couch!

MYTHS AND IDENTITIES: DO NOT EXPECT TOO MUCH FROM A GAME

According to Merriam-Webster, *myth* can be defined as "a usually traditional story of ostensibly historical events that serves to unfold part of the worldview of a people to explain a practice, belief, or natural phenomenon" (Merriam-Webster, 1989). A myth establishes shared beliefs of a community and rarely has any connection to the outside world. Contrary to popular belief, what we cannot put on the positive list for youth sports is evidence that sports reliably build "character" at any level of play. One great resource for more information on this subject is a book from Andrew Miracle and C. Roger Rees, *Lessons from the Locker Room* (1994). This book should be required reading for any parent or high school athletic director, as the lessons are timeless. In it they present a great deal of evidence and research against the "sports builds character" myth, and their conclusions were subsequently supported by multiple other studies (Camire & Trudel, 2010). As we say in psychology, these conclusions also hold up regarding "face validity." In other words, why would we think that sports build character more than any other team activity that requires effort? Would it build more character than working at Burger King? What about the Outdoor Club? Or playing in an orchestra? These are all activities that require cooperation and teamwork. Sports might often have the opposite effect, as many studies have shown (Miracle &

Rees, 1994). The goal of sports is not to keep the customer happy or make music. Children are sadly often taught the point of sports is to win, to be the highest scorer, to dominate the opposition. Now, winning can be a reasonable lesson if it is put in the right context and presented by knowledgeable, caring adults. Just as I allude to in the athlete-nonathlete dichotomy, we can strive to win as long as we are not teaching that the only other option is to *lose*. Respect for your opponent, just like respect for the effort in PE and in sports, needs to be the take-home lesson.

Part of the myth is that somehow school sports were key to the United States becoming an economic and military superpower, although quantifying such an abstraction is difficult and lacking data (O'Hanlon, 1983). Similarly, there are no good studies to support the myth that children who participate in sports are more successful than others because they learn "superiority" on the athletic field (Hyman, 2012). Some nonmythical positive aspects of youth sports is that while participating children generally eat better, take on fewer risky behaviors such as smoking, doing drugs, and having sex, and have fewer psychological issues (Pate et al., 2000). Those who play sports show no difference in drinking behavior, which might not be too much of a surprise considering the strong advertising relationship between sports and alcohol. Alas, these benefits are generally short-lived for the majority of young athletes, as this healthy behavior is not sustained after they stop playing. This is key, since by the time students reach high school, only about 15% to 50% are participating in sports (Pratt & Brody, 2014; Robert Wood Johnson Foundation, 2019). So what about some other benefits? We would all hope that sports participation would lead to developing lifelong friends, but the data supporting this are mostly anecdotal (Partridge, 2015). Ideally, organized sports can provide a forum for meeting children (and families) from different racial and socioeconomic backgrounds, helping fight prejudice. Who did not get goosebumps the first time they heard the story of Pee Wee Reese putting his arm around Jackie Robinson, not just to show the fans, but his teammates and the opposing team, that Jackie Robinson was his friend and equal? This is the purity of sports that we commonly see now only in the youngest competitors.

Measuring the effect of organized youth sports on social issues is understandably difficult to dissect as there is a large inherent bias. As noted, organized sports are more accessible to white, suburban households with generally a higher socioeconomic level than many inner-city or rural families. Thus when doing these studies, we are automatically looking at an already privileged group who have self-selected. Youth participation in sports requires parents with the interest, time, and wherewithal to register the children and support them regarding transportation, uniform costs, and more. A recent study from two economists at the IZA Institute of Labor Economics supports this concept of selection bias (Ransom & Ransom, 2018). They begin the study by defining "athletes" as "those who report having participated in 'athletics, cheerleading, or pep clubs' in high school" (again, the athlete/nonathlete divide). The authors go on to explain why they are evaluating this subject, noting:

> Sports are thought to be beneficial to youth because they provide a forum to develop important skills whose development otherwise tends to be omitted from traditional education. These skills include teamwork, persistence, patience, time management, and leadership skills. Furthermore, sports participation may be beneficial by increasing access to higher education through athletic scholarships, keeping troubled youth off the streets, matching youth with coaches who serve as mentors, and teaching youth proper health, physical fitness, and conditioning habits. . . . On the other hand, sports participation may be harmful to youth if it distracts too much from academic pursuits, if it causes excess physical injury, or if it encourages youth to spend more time with peers who are less academically inclined or more prone to risky behavior.

The authors' conclusions are consistent with those of almost all studies of their kind:

- Beneficial effects of sports have the noted "selection bias"—in other words, these children already had advantages, sports or no sports.
- The health benefits of playing organized sports were mixed, showing that men who played such sports in high school exercised in adulthood at a higher rate—but also, surprisingly, had a higher rate of obesity.
- They conclude with the lukewarm statement, "despite having very little human capital value, sports may still have a place in high school as a social or cultural activity" and paraphrase the sports commentator Heywood Hale Broun, who noted in 1974, "Sports do not build character; they reveal it."

THE ATHLETIC LOTTERY WINNERS

What is the purpose of our public schools? If a school's role is teaching a body of knowledge so children can grow into thoughtful, caring, inquisitive, healthy citizens, obtain jobs, and start lives on their own, then why is there such emphasis on competitive sports? Or, if sports are so important in teaching such values, then why are not all students required to participate? One could certainly assume sports are more important than academics by examining the school trophy case, signs on the roads into town, or banners hung over Main Street. Are there similar trophies, signs, and banners displayed for the Robotics Team state championship? Rarely. Yet scholarship is presumably what we are teaching and emphasizing in school and, if successful, should be a point of pride. As I tell my young patients, "You will make more money with your brains than you will with your legs"—and I have rarely been wrong. Too many students, and some members of the community, conflate participating in sports with receiving an education.

One relatively recent aspect of youth sports that I have witnessed during my career is this: The parent's goal for enrolling their child in various leagues is not necessarily for the children to play and have fun with their mates, but to get them to the "next level." This level could be a travel team, an "all-star" team, or simply the local high school team. ("You mean you didn't sign Alicia up for the U14 travel soccer squad? Kiss that college scholarship goodbye!") Often the move to the next level is not so much rooted in a child's interest or ability, but in the parents' willingness to put in the energy and money to make this happen. There is a huge amount of frightening information published discussing this subject (Gerdy, 2002; Miracle, 1994). The costs are so significant that it is not just the parents making the financial commitment. They often need help from other sources, especially relatives and community donations (Hyman, 2012). This latter "sponsorship" request is well known to the business owners in my own rural community, and it is the rare instance where they do not answer the call whether for individual players or teams. Although this works out if you happen to be living in the right place, it is less often an option for those in poor or economically disadvantaged areas. But again, this arrangement is generally in the early years of competition. Once a child reaches their middle and high school years, the entire district is obliged to be involved financially through their taxes. Though this arrangement solves one problem—family income is not as significant a factor for participation—it creates others. First, unless children have been playing organized league sports in their elementary years, they often lack the skill level to be anything but a bench player in high school (remember, few children are playing pickup games on their own these days). Second, sports do not further the child's academic achievement on the same level as aggressive PE classes. Third, with fewer than half of the students participating in high school sports, this chunk of money is being given to a minority of the student population.

Before going any further, let me be clear: I am not at all opposed to organized sports. I played little league, high school, and college sports (albeit poorly!). I appreciate the multiple benefits I received from participating, not realizing then I was gleaning these on the taxpayer's dime. The "athletic lottery winners," those children who already have strong physical identities, are the ones benefiting from our school sports system. Now, if your daughter is the best player on her AAU basketball team; if your family enjoys traveling to tournaments multiple weekends a year and you can absorb the expense; if she will be starring on the high school team and is already looking at potential college scholarships; I understand the guffaw. I get the fact that the system seems to be working—for you. With all due respect, until she gets those four years of State U paid for, finishes with healthy knees, and then finds a satisfying career, you might want to keep your head down. The chances of this happening, as you know, are staggeringly small. When you hit the lottery, all the money you spent on buying those tickets is worth it. But such winners are few. And similar to the way that low-income people subsidize the lottery where the money would probably be better spent elsewhere, your daughter's high school and college athletic "careers" (note I did not say "education") are being subsidized by the taxpayers of your town and state. My belief is it should not be the school's job to provide your daughter with a venue to play sports. It should be the school's job to have her *ready* to play sports.

One other potentially negative aspect of organized sports is a topic I will not dwell on despite my background as a sports medicine doctor and surgeon: injury risk. Remember, if I had my way, children would spend more time playing outside, finding adventure in the woods, on the streets, and in the water. If such were the case, there would certainly be more injuries than if they were playing video games. Luckily, when there is no whistle involved, children generally titrate the amount of risk they are willing to take, and there are fewer injuries than in organized sports. The risk of injury from outdoor activity does not deter me as a physician from recommending it, with the caveat that we eliminate any head contact. The positive aspects of motion, exercise, skills, and fun, both physical and psychological, are still much healthier than *not* being active, despite the injury risk (O'Neill, 2012).

There is another philosophical problem with supporting organized school sports teams as opposed to daily PE for all students that was alluded to earlier. If we accept that these sports are crucial to a child's development, why are we not insisting that everyone participate in them? And if everyone *should* be participating, that means everyone *needs* to participate—not six players seeing 90% of the minutes in a basketball game, but rotating everyone in equally. This model does exist in some private schools, but not in any public school to my knowledge. If we are to use sports for physical activity, for PE, it needs to be someone's job to ensure *every* child is on the move, is on the field, is *playing*—every day.

WILD GAME

When we discuss organized sports, the elephant in the room for many communities is American football. Football is an exciting but dangerous sport that is not only the most expensive, but does not allow participation of half of the school population, with rare exception. What of the fact that the Friday or Saturday football game gets back to that notion of national identity? Fair enough. Sports, and most especially football, are cultural phenomena, but they do not need to be tied to education. Here are just a few benefits of taking football out of the public schools and making it a community club sport:

- There is precedent for youth teams not being represented by a school but by a locale. This was how teams were established in the 1800s and into the 1900s before they came under the banner of the local school district and the influence of the sports-industrial complex. This is still the case in the elementary school–age children with Pop Warner. Also, there is good precedent around the world for community control of sports. A great example of this is the Gaelic Athletic Association (GAA) in Ireland.

- It would take the average person out of subsidizing something they might not support ethically (e.g., gender bias or concussion risk), or something that is not having a tangible benefit to the majority of students.
- It would eliminate the debate that has been going on since the beginning of school sports—that of conflating sports with education.
- Football is already on the wane. Although for decades we have accepted injuries to knees and shoulders, these usually will not change the arc of someone's life. This cannot be said about concussions and other head trauma incurred at a higher percentage in American football than any other sport (Stanford Children's Health, n.d.). A decrease in the numbers of children playing tackle football is already being seen as parents are understandably nervous about possible long-term health effects (Cook, 2019). As a result, football teams for many smaller schools are seeing fewer bodies, increasing the playing time and thus the injury risk of the remaining athletes. I suspect in the coming years the legal liability alone will make fielding a football team too expensive for many school budgets. However, I am all for keeping a community or county football program if that is what people want to support.

As a student or parent, you will ideally reap benefits from engagement in any school social activity, but with the help of the sports-industrial complex, competitive athletics has secured its own category in our cultural identity. When we discuss football, multiple images that are essentially cultural come to mind: the Super Bowl, New Year's Day, and of course the television series *Friday Night Lights*. Remember though, there is weak data at best to support the benefits of school sports, including football, any more than there is for band or drama club (Miracle, 1994). Despite this fixation, there seems to be a concern that by making such support for athletics voluntary at the club level, people might lose interest. Basically, they are saying that if every citizen is not forced to contribute to the team through their taxes, the sport will lose its popularity as it will cease to be "their" team, losing a "cultural touchstone." This simply does not make sense. All over the world, and originally in the United States, organized sports are part of the *community*, not part of an educational institution, and they are supported. The same will happen again in the United States if our system reverted to that of community control instead of school control.

THE RIGHT SIDE OF HISTORY

So how does this all relate to the problem at hand: students' health? Physical education by definition is a combination of physical and social science. If presented well, a good PE program has been shown empirically to pay dividends on both fronts: physical fitness, of course, but also social constructs of well-being, self-esteem, and academic performance for all students. Sports, including football, presumably promote a menu of societal benefits, including codes of behavior, conformity, productivity, fairness, cooperation, independence, and teamwork, but unfortunately there is no scientific data to support this. I appreciate that there is a reasonably large cohort of people out there who disagree with some of the changes I recommend (many being friends and family!). Athletic lottery winners who go on to college scholarships will be leading this disagreement cohort, though at some point we must as a society get on the right side of history. Although the present system may have worked on some levels historically, we are really talking about 100 years ago—not today.

Youth sports are strongly influenced by what we have been referring to as the sports-industrial complex (Maguire, 2006). In his book *The Case Against Sugar,* Gary Taubes (2018) presents a convincing discussion of the similarities between the tobacco and sugar industries. Mr. Taubes believes that tobacco and sugar were "separated at birth," but could we make a similar argument to include the sports industry? The sugar industry, similar to the sports industry, has managed an elaborate bait and switch. In the case of sugar, they have found another villain. "No, the problem is not sugar, it's fat—fat is your enemy! Fat makes people fat!" In the case of sports, multiple influences, to their own financial gain, have effectively switched school physical activity to sporting events.

There is denial regarding the impact on health from both the sugar industry and the sports industry. We have been sold sugar as being a good "energy food," just as we are sold sports as being good for health. Both can be true, but with a load of caveats. Many of the people in charge of youth sports sell their products as a part of healthy living, when in fact they are most often selling entertainment. If they were concerned with health, they would be promoting equal participation for all children, not being in the business of winning and creating icons. It would be my contention that the sports-industrial complex would ultimately make more money by not excluding the 75% of the population, but that might be another discussion. Michelle Obama understandably did not want to demonize the food industry when she introduced her "Let's Move" campaign, but maybe it is time to hold some people accountable in the food and sports industries for how they are marketing their products to our youngsters.

WHAT'S SO FUNNY 'BOUT PEACE, LOVE, AND UNDERSTANDING?

The original role of public school athletic programs was to support the financial progress and success of our society as a whole. The leaders of these movements were planning ahead to when the students would eventually be needed as workers and soldiers, and competitive sports were felt to support this need. But that was then. We no longer need workers for their brute strength or allegiance to a new government, but we do need workers not suffering from diabetes, obesity, dynapenia, depression, and the other maladies of humans who have lost their physical identities. We need at least a basic level of fitness to maintain a bright and agile mind. With the increase in these diseases, not only will it be more and more difficult to find enough young people fit enough for the military and the few physical jobs that remain, but today's youth might not have the physical stamina to keep up with a job in technology. Now that the role of physical activity affecting mental acuity is clear, we are not exercising for the plow, but we should be exercising for possible hours spent programming and innovating!

If we are playing sports to combat the health crisis, to build character, and to establish physical identity into adulthood, it is not working. Generally, if a behavior is driven by extrinsic motivation—in this case by parents and other adults often enrolling their children in these activities—it will rarely continue long term. Despite the discussion above, I believe there is great value in sports, but adults are often ruining the experience as shown by the number of children and early teens turning away from sports and flocking to video games. We need youngsters to be *intrinsically* motivated, which is simply allowing their primitive brain to work. They want to play. We must provide the venues and encouragement to let them.

Organized sports, with its built-in coaches/mentors, should be a place where we learn to follow established rules and get satisfaction from effort, no matter the outcome. In sport psychology we discuss "task orientation" and "goal orientation." If you are task oriented, you enjoy the process of learning, practicing, seeing improvement, and competing with your friends, no matter what the outcome. You are intrinsically motivated to play. If you are goal oriented, you are focused on the end result: winning. You are extrinsically motivated. Someone goal oriented and extrinsically motivated will eventually see defeat and then risk losing interest, the worst possible result.

A minor rebellion against organized sports has spawned many of the "extreme" sports. Mountain bikers, skateboarders, snowboarders, ultimate frisbee, and yes, even video gamers, felt alienated from more mainstream sports with their adult and corporate influences, and pioneered a whole new world of entertainment. Although video games in particular are hardly free of the sports-industrial complex influence, they are free of adult supervision. When children abandon organized sports, they look for another activity to fill their time. The ones with some physical identity take to the woods and streets on skis and bikes. For those with no physical identity, the easiest place to land is on their butts, right in front of a waiting screen.

Our children are growing up in a different world than we did. We must acknowledge this and make appropriate adjustments so they can become healthy, happy adults. Sports were meant to be a fun diversion, not a forum for character building, lessons in citizenship, and education. Once sports were found to generate jobs and big money for the sports-industrial complex, like so many things, they became a source of abuse. Shame on us for letting sports establish themselves as an integral part of, and often eclipsing, our education institutions' main role. Companies like Dick's Sporting Goods, a major sponsor of sporting events, do some brilliant charitable work, but at the end of the day they are there to generate profits. The job of Dick's is not to concern themselves with children's overall health or their learning geometry. I am not here to vilify Dick's or Nike or Under Armour— they are all trying to produce superior products and make money for their stockholders. As educators, we have a different calling. In a perfect world with unlimited time and money, perhaps we could have it all: daily PE, art, music, science, foreign languages, sports, history, and so on. *My job as a doctor, and I would submit the job of all adults, is to deliver our youth to the age of 18 healthy with their physical identity intact, understanding their part in the natural world around them.* If getting young people there includes organized sports, all the better, but it is more important regarding physical identity to develop a foundation of fitness without the competition factor (Friedman, 2013).

DON'T BECOME WHAT YOU EAT

I would be remiss without a short discussion regarding the horrible foods our children are eating. I emphasize throughout the book that our lifestyles have changed drastically over the past 50 years. The foods we eat have been a big part of this shift. As someone who has always been active but is taking daily medications for high blood pressure, I consider myself a victim of these dietary changes. To say the main cause of hypertension is due to genetics is letting ourselves off the hook. The evolution and availability of unnatural, ultra-processed foods are a major contributor to our health crisis. The definition of ultra-processed foods is one of those things that needs to be seen in its entirety to appreciate. Here you go:

> Industrial formulations typically with 5 or more and usually many ingredients. Besides salt, sugar, oils, and fats, ingredients of ultra-processed foods include food substances not commonly used in culinary preparations, such as hydrolyzed protein, modified starches, and hydrogenated or interesterified oils, and additives whose purpose is to imitate sensorial qualities of unprocessed or minimally processed foods and their culinary preparations or to disguise undesirable qualities of the final product, such as colorants, floorings, non-sugar sweeteners, emulsifiers, humectants, sequestrants, ad firming, bulking, de-foaming, anticaking, and glazing agents. (Gibney, 2019)

Certainly, the above would not be anything our great-grandparents would recognize as food, but these products are not going away, and thus we have to find a way to mitigate their effects. *By maintaining our physical identity, we will instinctively make better choices regarding food, activity, screen time, and numerous other health options.* I ask my patients each New Year's Eve to enact small health changes, as these will add up over time. Get the ultra-processed and sugar-laden foods out of the pantry. Make organic choices where possible. Buy local foods that are not just better for you, but better for the environment. Maintain a predominantly plant-based diet. Cook and eat meals together as a family. Discourage snacking in general, but perhaps give the option of some cut-up fruit or an apple—if the healthy choice is *easy*, we will usually take it.

We read to our children, we dress them in warm clothes, we immunize them (please), we make changes in our buildings to eliminate lead paint and asbestos, so why in the world would we expose them to large quantities of toxic food filled with antibiotics and preservatives? I am not naive and have fond memories of that package of Hostess CupCakes I occasionally scored as a child. But such "treats" were few and far between. Even 50 years ago parents understood this was not something to be consumed on a regular basis if you wanted your child to grow up healthy. Serving good food is part of raising a child. If finances for healthy choices are an issue, there are programs in most communities to help. We do not smoke around our children. Allowing access to unlimited amounts of high-calorie, low-nutrient foods is the equivalent of having them grow up in a cigar bar.

REBRANDING

Finally, I used a word multiple times: rebranding. According to Professor Niall Moyna, one of the problems with PE is it is stuck in the 19th century and needs rebranding for the changes in the 21st. We will discuss in the coming chapters what this actually could look like in practice, but what should we call it? New or "enhanced" physical education? (Personally, I think we need to eliminate anything with these last two words as they carry too much baggage.) How about Fast-time? PlayFast? MoveTime? Motion Class? Kid-time? Motion Learning? Learn Time? Happy and Fit? Fitness Class? Running (the "fourth R"). Or maybe it is not my job to overthink the room. Perhaps we should bring in the thoughts of Silicon Valley, as they are a big part of what has us in this mess. They have managed to sell unhealthy, addictive products to our children—let us ask them to sell something positive. Sell "Motion Class" as the favorite part of the day for every child—not something to dread—but something to help maintain their physical identity.

CHAPTER 3

Roadblocks to Rebranding Physical Education in Today's Schools

EXPERIENCE VS. EXPERTISE

Try watching the Super Bowl with a room full of ex–high school football players. Everyone is an expert and infinitely smarter than the coaches or referees on the field. The same hubris can be heard when discussing education. This is human nature but also speaks to the importance of the experience vs. expertise discussion earlier. All people have experience with education—they do not have *expertise*. As we say in the research business, you are an "n of one." In other words, while *your* experience was *your* experience and should be considered as a data point in a study, it is still only one data point.

We now have tons of data regarding climate change. Whatever weather patterns you have seen in your area of late, I am here to tell you that climate change is real. Do you know why? Because people who have spent years and years studying this subject have drawn those conclusions (Union of Concerned Scientists, 2018). There comes a time when we must listen to the experts unless we are willing to put in the time to become one ourselves. This is also why when I tell you the best treatment for your unstable knee ligament is reconstruction, you believe me. As an orthopedic surgeon, I am an expert on this subject, and I have the science to support my opinion.

Now that we have looked at some of the historical issues regarding physical education (PE), in this chapter we will examine the present state of PE in light of the latest research and expertise, and why we seem to struggle to make positive changes. Along the way I will continue to agitate for reforms that can be enacted *now*, with no significant financial burden to the taxpayers. If you have good memories of your PE experience, that will help my cause. If you have bad memories, perhaps there are some things we could agree on so the same will not be said by your children (our "rebranding"). PE is simply too important a class in today's world for students to hate.

If we plunked down doctors from 100 years ago in a university hospital today, they would be lost. New techniques based on a century of research would leave them far behind even a first-year medical student. But if pioneering experts in physical education such as Horace Mann, Dudley Sargent, Catherine Beecher, or Luther Gulick appeared in an elementary school gym class, they would be horrified at what was *not* happening and proceed to take over the class. Is there any other profession where we could say this? Muscle-strengthening techniques have not changed terribly over the past century, even allowing for fads to come and go. Yet these pioneers would be dismayed by the lack of urgency, intention, and simply time in most PE curricula today. This is not for want of expertise. This is due to lack of will on the part of those making PE decisions. It is due to apathy, cultural mores, and especially because "that's the way we have always done it" despite the extraordinary changes in the last 50 years. Similar to climate studies, there is almost universal consensus that children are not getting enough exercise. Agreeing there is a problem is a beginning—just how to address it is a bit stickier.

At the turn of the last century, if youngsters were not getting PE or playing sports in school, they were not lacking for activity. If children were not playing "pickup games" after school in 1900, they were working on the farm, in shops, delivering papers, caring for family, and, sadly, often working in factories. These responsibilities were not alternatives to today's activities; they were mandates: Unless you were wealthy, almost all children had to participate in the family economy for survival. Even for the laziest humans out there, there was no way to avoid a certain amount of physical activity. If one was rich enough to have a car, it was almost as labor intensive as a horse! What children were *not* doing in the early 1900s was sitting inside playing video games and eating fast food.

Many of us are guilty of thinking our ancestors were somehow ignorant because of what they believed and how they lived their lives. They prayed to gods for everything from rain to toothaches. They believed the world was flat. They thought women too weak to run a marathon (but never too weak to cook, harvest, and clean all day!). At the start of my own career, physicians believed patients with back pain should go to bed for three days. There were plenty of super smart people "back in the day," but they were simply working with the cultural knowledge base (and prejudices) of the times. Part of my job every day is to ask what I might be criticized for by young doctors 20 years from now. One thing we *cannot* criticize our ancestors for is not recognizing the importance of "physical education." I put this in quotes because PE has had different phases and forms but always pointed to the need for the human body to move (there's that primitive brain again). Motion of all types was indeed part of our culture.

PE in America started racing ahead at the turn of the last century, though it began almost as soon as public schools were being established in the mid-1800s. Much of the early PE was based on the German (Friedrich Jahn, Charles Beck) and Swedish (Pehr Ling) concepts of exercise (LeCorre, 2018), and some of the first indoor gymnastics equipment devised by these PE forerunners is still being used today. The English, as discussed, are credited for bringing competitive organized youth sports to our shores. Multiple founders of the PE movement, including Dudley A. Sargent, were medical doctors. When I was obtaining my education degree, I was reminded daily of Dr. Sargent, as his name still adorns the School of Health and Rehabilitation Sciences at Boston University. Dr. Sargent, who died in 1924, invented early versions of the machines you see in exercise clubs today, with multiple weights and pulleys (DelaPena, 2003). He was also one of the first to quantify progress in the gym by taking measurements and comparing these over time. Sargent, along with Catherine Beecher years before him, were strong advocates of women's fitness. It was Ms. Beecher who established the first-known program of calisthenics specifically for women at the Hartford (CT) Female Seminary in 1823 (The Editors of Encyclopaedia Britannica, 2019).

Health and hygiene, such as hair and teeth brushing, were a big part of the early PE "curriculum." This emphasis is perhaps not surprising as Louis Pasteur was proving his germ theory during this time period. In 1866, California, setting trends for the country even then, had the distinction of being the first state to legislate exercise *twice a day* for school children (Boyce, n.d.). PE was championed by no less an educational reformer than John Dewey, and by the early 1900s PE was established as a specialty in the field of education (ibid.). As a result, with the increasing number of "normal schools," or colleges that specifically educated teachers, PE became its own degree with substantial training in anatomy and physiology. By the early 1920s, most states had a PE requirement for public school students ("About SPARK", n.d.).

Looking at PE through a wide lens allows the appreciation of cultural patterns that have emerged over decades. Massachusetts became a state in 1788 and enacted compulsory public education in 1852 (though compulsory education technically started when under British rule in 1647!) ("Compulsory Education Laws: Background," 2016). In contrast, Mississippi became a state 29 years after Massachusetts (1817) but was the last in the nation to legislate compulsory public education 100 years later in 1917 (that's all education, not just PE) (ibid.). Despite many excellent minds and a strong state university, education was never made an important part of the culture in Mississippi, and that legacy continues to this day. Mississippi is 1 of 11 states to not fund prekindergarten education and consistently ranks toward the bottom in educational rubrics. On the other hand, Massachusetts historically valued public education and today scores toward the top in the United States in most public education assessments (Hess, 2018). Fortunately, as we will see later, Mississippi is making strides in PE, which will only help boost the state's academic standing. As emphasized many times in this book, the overall health of our nation depends on everyone making physical health an important part of the culture.

FEDERAL INPUT FOR PHYSICAL EDUCATION

The historic trend of emulating the English model of organized sports in public schools in favor of exercise for general fitness was in large part due to the influence of industry and the military (Betts, 1953). Industrial leaders in the early 1900s felt that team sports could be useful for developing citizens capable of working in factories and businesses. Initially, the military's interest in PE was not so much a concern regarding the fitness of thousands of new American immigrants, but more in their ability to understand the chain of command and follow orders. As the century proceeded, the pendulum swung back to the belief that the fitness of Americans was lagging behind that of our European counterparts, making us potentially vulnerable in times of war. The belief that Americans were unfit continued to wax and wane throughout the years, leading to multiple pushes for curriculum changes *from sports to fitness*. The bombing of Pearl Harbor in 1941 and the Kraus-Weber Minimum Fitness testing and reporting in the early 1950s helped to solidify these beliefs (Miller, n.d.). The next push from sports to fitness, and the one baby boomers will remember, was championed by President John F. Kennedy with the President's Council on Physical Fitness. The decline of such programs is another factor that has led to the current state of physical education in the nation's public schools.

In the late 1950s, partly due to the influence of Dr. Hans Kraus and his research, President Dwight Eisenhower believed there to be a decrease in the fitness of Americans in the years after World War II and the Korean War (Holland, 2018). Interestingly, the issues leading to poor fitness presented to President Eisenhower at that time were the same that we discuss today: a decrease in farm work, modernization of factories, and too much screen time (this was the dawn of TV). Although the President's Council of Physical Fitness was established in the late 1950s, it was not until President Kennedy took an interest that things really progressed. Though the federal government had no power to mandate a national fitness program, through savvy marketing and the use of the president's "bully pulpit," a core group of almost a quarter-million schoolchildren took part in the pilot project in six states (John F. Kennedy Library and Museum, n.d.). Improved student fitness was soon demonstrated, and the program went nationwide. I myself as a boy in the 1960s remember *trying* to pass this fitness test and receive the accompanying Presidential Certificate (with its significant social cache in the fifth-grade lunchroom!).

Physical fitness was a cornerstone and remains a legacy of the short-lived Kennedy administration. President Kennedy wrote eloquently on the subject in his "Progress Report by the President on Physical Fitness" (1963). In it, he compared the need for regular exercise in our own times with that of the ancient Romans and Greeks, who understood "it was necessary to have not only a free and inquiring mind, but a strong and active body to develop." In this same report, the president also tied fitness to "happiness," a word rarely heard in formal American discourse since the Declaration of Independence.

Since President Kennedy, the federal government's effort encouraging physical fitness has continued with various levels of enthusiasm. Star power has been a part of the council, involving such sports luminaries as Mariano Rivera. In 2010, President and Michelle Obama added "nutrition" as part of the council's purview, and soon after, Ms. Obama started the "Let's Move" campaign in 2012 (Executive Order 13545—President's Council on Fitness, Sports and Nutrition, 2010). The stated goal of the "Let's Move" initiative is to have students in all grades moving at least 60 minutes a day. Today, the President's Council on Fitness, Sports and Nutrition states that its mission is to empower "America to adopt a healthy lifestyle that includes regular physical activity and good nutrition" (ibid.).

The testing aspect of the council has produced an offshoot, the Presidential Youth Fitness Program. This was started in 2012, with the motto of "empowering students to be fit for life" (Presidential Youth Fitness Program, n.d.). The program continues to be voluntary and still includes a fitness assessment (though I am told the egalitarian badges do not create the same buzz as the old certificates). The program is weighted, however, more toward encouragement to adopt healthier living and health-related fitness. Now, these are all good things, and perhaps harken back to the hygiene training a century and a half earlier. However, there is some redundancy in these programs, and importantly they seem to lack the government effort the original council showed back in the 1960s. Once again it is this lack of urgency and intention regarding fitness, coupled with the increased urgency for teaching subjects requiring standardized testing, that is helping leave us in the place we are today regarding the nation's physical fitness.

PHYSICAL EDUCATION IN AMERICAN SCHOOLS TODAY

There are four questions we will attempt to answer in this section to give us a view of what a PE class looks like today in America:

Question 1: What are the evidence-based standards?
Question 2: What is happening state by state, and why are they so different?
Question 3: What are PE teachers being taught?
Question 4: Are we waist deep in the big muddy?

1: What Are the Evidence-Based Standards?

I would encourage the interested reader to avail themselves of a great resource on this topic: *Educating the Student Body: Taking Physical Activity and Physical Education to School,* published in 2013 by the National Academies Press (Institute of Medicine, 2013). This publication lays out the science behind their recommendations for PE across the nation. Most states acknowledge the scholarship establishing these standards, but few schools follow them, and this is to the detriment of our students. Similar to advising a patient with back pain to take to bed, not following the evidence-based research is, to my mind, educational malpractice.

Let us just start with some basics. According to *Educating the Student Body,* physical education can be defined as "a planned sequential K–12 standards-based program of curricula and instruction designed to develop motor skills, knowledge, behaviors of healthy active living, physical fitness, sportsmanship, self-efficacy, and emotional intelligence." They go on to state a proper PE program should:

- Be instructed by certified PE teachers.
- Comprise a minimum of 30 minutes a day for elementary school students and 45 minutes a day for middle and high schoolers.
- Set tangible standards for achievement, including for high school graduation.
- Advocate for binding requirements that address state standards, curriculum time, and class size.

The National Association of Sports and Physical Education (NASPE), an organization representing PE teachers, has in their *Instructional Framework for Fitness Education in Physical Education* specifics of what should be a part of every school's curriculum and the goal for every student:

a. **Technique:** Demonstrate competency in techniques needed to perform a variety of moderate to vigorous physical activities (MVPA).
b. **Knowledge:** Demonstrate understanding of fitness concepts, principles, strategies, and individual differences needed to participate and maintain a health-enhancing level of fitness.
c. **Physical activity:** Participate regularly in fitness-enhancing physical activity.
d. **Health-related fitness:** Achieve and maintain a health-enhancing level of health-related fitness.
e. **Responsible personal and social behaviors:** Exhibit responsible personal and social behaviors in physical activity settings.
f. **Values and advocates:** Value fitness-enhancing physical activity for disease prevention, enjoyment, challenge,

self-expression, self-efficacy, and/or social interaction and
allocate energies toward the production of healthy
environments.

g. **Nutrition:** Strive to maintain a healthy diet through
knowledge, planning, and regular monitoring.

h. **Consumerism:** Access and evaluate fitness information,
facilities, products, and services. (NASPE)

Clearly, the guidance is there on a *national* level. Let's take a deeper dive into some of these recommendations and see if we can understand why they are not being followed across the country at the
district level.

A Proper Program Should Be Instructed by Certified PE Teachers

The number of certified PE teachers in the United States exceeds
200,000 ("How to Become a Phys Ed Teacher," n.d.). This number is
not enough to cover the requirements of providing daily PE for all students. The same could be said about the shortage of doctors needed for
basic medical services. One of the solutions in medicine has been to
employ "midlevel" providers, such as physician's assistants and nurse
practitioners to fill the gaps. Just now, there are no such alternative
personnel commonly employed in the world of PE. However, "paraprofessionals" (i.e., PE teaching assistants) with the proper training
could attend to bureaucratic details and basic supervision, allowing
the certified PE teacher's time to be used more efficiently. A PE assistant's salary would also be significantly less than that of a certified
teacher (an average PE teacher costs about $120,000 once all benefits
are included, while a paraprofessional would cost less than half of
that) while providing an added resource to keep students moving and
safe. *The use of teaching assistants is a key component to my plan for our PE
revolution and will be discussed in more detail later in the book.*

A Proper Program Should Have a Minimum Daily Time for PE

The concept of daily, habit-forming activity is absolutely key to the
maintenance of physical identity. *We cannot let physical identity ever lapse,*
as it is terribly hard to gain back. Since the passage of the No Child Left
Behind Act in 2002, almost half of schools claim to have taken time
away from PE and recess to increase time in other subjects, especially

math and English (McMurrer, 2008). As noted when discussing the President's Council of Physical Fitness, physical education curricula are not within the purview of the federal government, and thus this is one of the reasons for the enormous differences from state to state, and even district to district. NASPE agrees with the need for *daily PE for all students,* and though it is the largest organization of PE teachers, it too can only give suggestions and guidelines. Ultimately, it is up to the school districts to model (or not) their particular programs to fit *any* standards. This is because even though there might be national or state standards, actual mandates and oversight are essentially nonexistent. The recent virus pandemic shined a light onto how much responsibility is on our school systems. Sadly, physical identity is another burden that must be taken on for the health of children going forward.

A PE teacher responds:

> At some point, families should take responsibility for making sure that their children are active (it doesn't have to be structured sports/activities). As teachers, an awful lot of responsibility to "fix" a child is put on us.

Since the amount of time to educate students in all subjects is limited, in order for PE to compete there needs to be a sense of *urgency.* A seventh grader might become interested in arithmetic if they find an inspiring teacher, and go on to a career as a mathematician. In contrast, once a child's physical identity is lost in kindergarten, first, or second grade, this identity can be lost forever, especially considering that in many schools the students have the same PE teacher for years. Once a child is labeled "unmotivated" or worse, a "nonathlete," it is human nature for the teacher to assume they will not change. But of course, at the elementary level, these incredibly impressionable and malleable young people absolutely *can* change. Maybe they need a new setting or a different activity or some extra help, but they are not finished with physical learning, any more than they are finished reading James Joyce. The effort required at later stages to establish physical identity once it is lost is much greater than the effort needed to improve academically (Blomain et al., 2013). Though a mediocre student in high school, my academic interests peaked in college and my grades followed suit. Anyone who has tried to regain fitness after years of overeating and not exercising knows the difficulty of this undertaking, and perhaps would prefer the challenge of quantum mechanics!

A Proper Program Should Have Tangible Standards Including for High School Graduation

We expect good teaching to result in increased student achievement. Determining what, if any, PE achievement standards one needs to establish is no easy matter. *Educating the Student Body* presents a framework for achievement based on current research and literature. Although all states have set standards for measuring what children should be learning or achieving in PE, similar to the setup of the PE program itself, the extent to which students achieve the goals is questionable as no accountability is required. (Iowa was the last holdout in setting state standards, adopting them in 2019 [State Board of Education Adopts New Physical Education, Health Standards for Iowa Schools, 2019].) Why, as with Common Core Standards, (it's not good to grind your teeth teachers!), there are no consequences for schools that do not help their students live a healthy lifestyle, is hard to understand. "Health" can be measured in many ways—but someone needs to hold a school's feet to the fire to at least make some headway. We will discuss just the person who can do this a bit later in this chapter.

Measuring or any other testing of "tangible PE standards" is a controversial subject and best left to the local PE professional, but someone needs to be collecting data. If we do not collect data of some kind, how do we know any program is working? We should at least be taking an "exercise vital sign" from our students to give some gauge of their physical activity (Faigenbaum & Bruno, 2017). Although our certified PE teachers have the background in math and science to understand and interpret the results of any physical testing, bringing in the classroom teachers, as well as the students themselves, would be an easy cross-discipline lesson. When available (and I hesitate to say this), they can enlist the student's smartphone technology to measure health indices, not just to provide entertainment.

That said, I do not think quantifying achievement standards has to be terribly complicated. The school nurse and local pediatricians could potentially get involved for measurements such as body mass index (BMI), but *effort and fun* in PE class are to my mind the needed outcomes. Once a school *commits to everyday PE that keeps their students in motion for 30+ minutes*, the results will soon be obvious. The only absolutely necessary data the school must collect should be comments from staff and visitors on the increased energy level, better test scores, and positive attitudes of the students. The other obvious "data point" should be reports from the parents that their children just seem . . . happier! Much of the depression in our society stems from trying to be something we are not. We were not born to be couch potatoes. We are primitive hunter-gatherers that need to be physical for true contentment. Dogs are not happy unless they get to run wild and explore. Humans are no different.

Setting standards for high school graduation can take many forms, with ample room for imagination. Motivated juniors and seniors are certainly capable of leading outdoor activities they have a passion for, and passing on that passion to the younger students. Programs could take the form of hiking trips incorporating plant and animal identification, mountain bike rides with same, walking trips to a local museum or historic site—basically, anything that involves getting up, moving, learning, and having fun away from a screen. The older students might receive PE credits toward graduation, knowing there is no better way to learn than to teach.

A Proper Program Should Advocate for Binding Requirements That Address State Standards, Curriculum Time, and Class Size

To this point we have been discussing aspirations for PE from national bodies—the President's Council, the National Academies Press, as well as criteria for a proper PE program presented by the NASPE. But, of course, these are *national* organizations that have no credentials to make change at the state, much less school district level. The approach used by school districts to fulfill a PE requirement will vary depending on who is making the decisions and if they have any interest in following state or national standards or "advocate for binding requirements."

State standards have evolved because our world has changed dramatically in the last 50 years. Many of us remember being given a pile of balls and bats in gym class and being hustled outside. This actually might be fine for high schoolers with some motivation and leadership, as it was for my classmates and me in the 1970s (nobody questioned John Walsh!). Most children, however, need a bit more direction and supervision. If the local PE teachers do not have the belief and skill to keep their students engaged and moving, positive change simply will not happen. Unfortunately, it is the rare administrator who will challenge the teaching methods of their PE teachers. For that, we need someone who has no rear-view mirror, but will be passionate for the way PE can and should be. What we need is a *"PE czar."*

A new process for ensuring accountability in following best practices is necessary, and toward that end I suggest that each state appoint a P.E. czar. The czar would see to existing resources being up to date and utilized, to new resources being made available, and to students getting the activity they need. The appointment of a czar places the onus of accountability on the place where the standards are conceived: the state capital.

The job of the czar will not be easy, but it will be influential. I envision this job as an appointment by the state secretary of education, and thus it will have immediate gravitas. The czar would have low pay but high prestige, ideal for someone with multiple contacts toward the end of a career in education. Similar to the President's Council on Physical Fitness, the czar will enlist local community leaders for their insight, ideas, and help at the district level. Successful communities could then assist/advise other communities at no cost—roles similar to serving on the boards of local charities.

The czar will importantly wield his or her influence regarding curriculum time. Although I appreciate these are issues that plague every teacher (classroom or specials), daily PE has to be the anchor of the schedule as a fitter child will be a better learner in all subjects. Czars will have the ear of the secretary of education and the governor, and in addition to their other duties, will go beyond most state standards by leading the campaign to mandate PE for every child, every day, in every district.

A classroom teacher responds:

When it comes to academics, standardized testing seems the only emphasis these days. You now bring up the other buzzword in education today, "time." The message that we need physical fitness for academic fitness I have never heard mentioned. One attempt to integrate different disciplines into the curriculum that has seen some success is writing. We ask the students to explain math with language and write about scientific concepts. There are programs such as "Read Across America" where for a week, at multiple times during the school day everything stops and the students read for 10 minutes. Of course, even this was difficult to schedule but like anything, if the leadership is there and the importance is understood, it should succeed. I think a similar program could work with movement and exercise. But what class or program will give up their time? That is the real challenge.

2: What Is Happening State by State, and Why Are We So Different?

Definitions of PE vary, but they all use the words "physical" and "education," as well as often incorporating concepts like "health," "lifelong," "skills," and "movement." There seems to be little argument about the general importance of PE. A recent survey from The Society of Health and Physical Educators found that 91% of parents also understood the need for PE and actually wanted more for their children (SHAPE America Society of Health and Physical Educators, n.d.). However, as noted, there is simply no consistency even across schools in the same district, of what PE should actually look like. When, how much, and what form PE should take is where the real disagreements come. For example, only six states require PE in every grade. According to the CDC, only 4% of elementary students had *daily* PE, while only 2% of high school students had such a requirement (CDC, 2020). Almost 70% of elementary schools have a PE requirement, but 20% of elementary schools allow exemption from PE for various nonmedical reasons, including participation in band or chorus. To make matters worse, in some school districts, students can take PE *online*! I suspect this has President Kennedy rolling over in his grave. Finally, a significant percentage of PE is taught by classroom teachers or others not trained specifically for this subject.

Statements regarding such variations could go on and on, with nothing of this sort being able to be said about teaching reading or math, particularly in the schools that adhere to the Common Core Standards. The one thing we can say about PE instruction in our schools is that it is "consistently inconsistent." But how does this happen when there is good science supporting evidence-based standards? First, there is no federal *mandate*—we only detailed above what could be thought of as recommended *standards*. Second, the state standards rarely follow the evidence-based standards. Third, as discussed earlier, there are no state *mandates* or oversight. Even if a mandate were in place, many schools would not follow them barring any consequences for not doing so.

Examples of State Standards

On state websites, there is often great detail regarding what they believe a child should be learning in PE class at each stage of development.

These standards are usually well meaning and appropriately researched by professionals. I would encourage the reader to do an Internet search of their own state standards, as well as neighboring states, to appreciate the wide variability in these documents. For the purpose of comparison, we will hone in only on the *time standard*, as I firmly believe that is where a school must start before any real progress can be made. As *Educating the Student Body* concludes, the evidence-based data recommends a minimum of *30 minutes a day for elementary school and 45 minutes a day for middle and high schoolers*. Let's see what some different states aspire to. We picked on California, Mississippi, and Massachusetts before, so let's stay with those three. We will also add my own state of New Hampshire, and a state who claims to be a "positive outlier," Illinois, as other examples and to cover the country.

California: California became a state in 1850. According to the *Physical Education Model Content Standards for California Public Schools, Kindergarten Through Grade Twelve* that was adopted by the California State Board of Education in 2005 and reposted in 2010, the state has backed off a bit from the "twice daily" exercise suggested in 1866 (Physical Education Model Content Standards for California, 2017). Today, a California elementary school student should have "three to four days each week in moderate to vigorous physical activities (MVPA) that increase breathing and heart rate" and by middle school this is a firm 4 days a week. High school students should participate in "moderate to vigorous physical activity at least four days each week" but only need to do this for 2 of the 4 years of high school. Another 2 years of PE would be considered "elective."

The state is careful not to be too draconian in making recommendations, a position followed by the California Department of Education (CDE) *Physical Education Model Content Standards*:

> Standards-based education maintains California's tradition of respect for local control of schools. To help students achieve at high levels, local educators—with the full support and cooperation of families, businesses, and community partners—are encouraged to apply these standards and design the specific curricular and instructional strategies that best deliver the content to their students. . . . The model content standards provide opportunities for teachers to reinforce student learning in all areas of the curriculum.

The CDE goes on to say something that warms my heart: "The standards link the content in PE with content in English–language arts, science, mathematics, and history–social science, *thereby establishing and emphasizing the many connections between the subjects*" (italics mine).

This kind of language gets me excited, and as I grade this website, it goes up with this statement. The CDE does not, however, hit the time suggestions recommended by the literature; thus I give California PE standards a grade of "B."

Mississippi: Mississippi, due to its checkered history of compulsory education and its present socioeconomic status, has a big hole to dig out of. That said, their website mentions many of the right things regarding PE. The Mississippi Department of Education published a document titled *The 2013–2014 Mississippi Physical Education Framework*, which provides standards for use by all PE instructors (Mississippi Department of Education, n.d.). The document goes on to note that the "Mississippi Healthy Students Act" passed by the state legislature requires "150 minutes of physical education/physical activity each week for students in grades K–8 and a 1/2 Carnegie Unit for graduation for grades 9–12." (A Carnegie Unit is 120 hours of class time with an instructor over the course of a year.) In a 36-week academic year, this would roughly equate to attending half a year of PE, the same requirement as California, though taken over 4 years instead of 2. The 150 minutes-a-week requirement hits the standard for elementary but falls short of the standard for middle schoolers.

The added value Mississippi notes on its Department of Education website is the involvement of outside agencies such as Project Fit America and the Blue Cross & Blue Shield Foundation of Mississippi. For this type of forward thinking and a decent elementary time commitment, I give the Mississippi standards a grade of "B+."

Massachusetts: The *Massachusetts Comprehensive Health Curriculum Framework*, published online by the Massachusetts Department of Education in 1999, is an extraordinary document of over 100 pages. The document goes into amazing detail regarding a host of health and PE-related topics. There is an *expectation* of physical education K–12, but I could not find specific time standards (I will hold my tongue on the use of the word "expectation"). In fact, Massachusetts does not require specific curricula or regulations enforcing time and student participation requirements for physical education. Thus, the decisions are made by the local school districts, which may or may not work to the students' advantage.

Massachusetts's grade improves with the statement "A major component of comprehensive school health education is parental and family involvement." This speaks to the vital topic of culture and physical identity. Unfortunately, the document goes on to say that "The state has an education report card for each school, but physical education is not included as one of the subject areas." This is unacceptable as we know the potential value of PE in these times. Massachusetts's heart seems to be in the right place, but they give the individual schools too much leeway; I give them a grade of "C."

New Hampshire: I include New Hampshire in this review as it is a small state and home to many fine private "college prep" high schools that served as a model for our current public system. New Hampshire is also home to Plymouth State University, a school that started life as The Plymouth Normal School in 1871. "Normal" meaning their teacher graduates were meant to "instill and reinforce particular norms." As the institution evolved into its present identity, it became a leader in training teachers, including those in PE (Plymouth State University). The other reason I chose to include New Hampshire is that it happens to be my home.

The *New Hampshire K–12 Physical Education Curriculum Guidelines* states that its purpose is to "provide a vision for physical education in New Hampshire" (New Hampshire Department of Education, 2005). It goes on to say that the "expectations for student learning at . . . levels set forth in this document are to be used as a *tool for districts*, schools and teachers to make *local decisions* about a comprehensive physical education curriculum" (italics mine). In other words, similar to our neighbor to the south, New Hampshire allows the school district to make the rules. The only quantitative statement is that "children should participate in a minimum of sixty minutes of physical activity daily," but the document does not specify the form of that activity or how it should happen.

There are many things I did like about these well-written curriculum guidelines. They admit to the obesity issue as well as the link between physical activity and cognition, stating:

[P]hysical education remains one of the student's primary sources for obtaining information on making informed decisions regarding one's lifestyle as it relates to physical activity as well as preventing life threatening diseases such as obesity and diabetes. . . . Obesity, high blood pressure and diabetes have increased significantly in the American population over the last decade. In this current health crisis, physical education as part of the regular school curriculum is critical . . . physical education offered in schools stimulates brain function, which increases focus and memory that results in students performing better academically.

We know that according to the CDC, the childhood obesity rate is around 20%—not just "overweight," but "obese" (National Center for Chronic Disease Prevention and Health Promotion, 2018). That means almost one in five children you see on the playground is obese.

Despite discussing the global issues of obesity and learning associated with PE, the New Hampshire guidelines give the schools too many outs, and thus only gets a grade of "C."

Illinois: I choose Illinois as our final state example for two reasons. First, we needed a representative from the middle of the country, and second, Illinois is said to have the strictest requirements of any state.

In the *Illinois Enhanced Physical Education Strategic Plan*, published in 2012, Illinois claims to be the first state in the nation to require daily PE for all students (Illinois State Board of Education, 2012). Although there might be some semantics to argue, Illinois does have a 30-minute-per-day requirement for kids K–6, similar to Mississippi. Perhaps the most impressive aspect of the Illinois State Board of Education's strategic plan is the recognition of the problem and the commitment to enacting positive changes. In fact, Illinois is brutally honest regarding the problem, stating:

The impact sedentary lifestyles are having on Illinois children is alarming. In 2007, a national survey on children's health showed that only three states—Mississippi, Georgia, and Kentucky—had a higher childhood obesity rate than Illinois. This means children in Illinois are at excessive risk for serious lifelong health problems like diabetes, heart disease, high cholesterol, and arthritis. . . . A sedentary lifestyle not only imperils the health of kids, it also threatens our economic future, which could make funding public education and other critical services even more challenging than ever before. A growing body of research suggests that obesity is largely to blame for our ballooning healthcare costs. Right now, 7.5% of all healthcare costs are spent on the treatment of chronic diseases, many of which are obesity-related. Obesity is a rapidly escalating problem that costs the Illinois health care system and taxpayers nearly $4 billion per year—including more than $1 billion to Medicaid and $800 million to Medicare annually. Some experts predict that, if nothing changes, the cost of obesity to the Illinois health care system will increase to $14 billion a year by 2018.

Wow. But with as cold an eye as Illinois puts on the obesity crisis, they do not end there. Just because a child is physically in a gym class, they still might not be getting significant physical exercise. Referring again to the literature, the Illinois strategic plan states:

> Unfortunately, physical activity times in P.E. classes are consistently low. Activity time in a traditional P.E. class can be less than 37% of the total class time. In a typical 30-minute (K–6 grade) class, students engage in only 11 minutes of physical activity. Thus, a traditional P.E. class contributes very little to ensuring students are meeting the 60 minutes per day of exercise recommended in the Physical Activity Guidelines for Americans (U.S. Department of Health and Human Services, 2008).

And this is followed by even more brutal honesty. The plan's authors also admit that some of the poorer schools are simply not on the same level as others, stating:

> There are also many schools who do not offer P.E. classes at all. According to the 2009 Youth Risk Behavior Survey, among Chicago high school students, "40% did not attend physical education (P.E.) classes in an average week when they were in school. Sixty percent did not attend P.E. classes daily when they were in school."

After this honest assessment, Illinois then discusses solutions, introducing the "enhanced P.E. program." This program commits to daily PE for K–12, increased activity while in class, wellness programs, funding commitments, teacher development, and community involvement. The authors state a goal to not only deal with childhood obesity, but to "promote academic achievement and realize the lifetime benefits of fitness" and "to prevent adult-onset obesity as well."

Finally, the plan introduces something that we as a nation have done successfully with drunk driving, though not at all successfully with gun violence. Illinois defines obesity and lack of activity as a "public health issue. School nurses and the school health system should be included on the front lines of this initiative." This type of forward thinking is brilliant.

The crisis of American fitness has been presented in various forms for decades, with real progress actually achieved in the early 1960s, when we as a nation acknowledged it. Again, there are few disagreements about the problem. The rub remains the solution. Illinois seems to be moving in the right direction. I give their strategic plan a rare "A." They have a good feel for the problem and have proposed a solution. Now for the implementation—and in that I wish them luck, and encourage them to read Chapter 5!

Roadblocks to Change

So what are some of the "roadblocks" ("barriers") keeping us from implementing these changes? *Educating the Student Body* gives a fairly exhaustive list of "Barriers to the Delivery of Physical Education," breaking things down to "Institutional," "Teacher-Related," and "Student-Related."

Under "Institutional," not surprisingly, the issues were predominantly facilities (infrastructure), which translates to *money*. Also not surprisingly, "time" is on every list. Easier to correct than a lack of money and time but also high on the list are administration and staff support. Other institutional barriers are large class size, number of PE staff, and lack of professional development.

Under the category of "Teacher-Related" barriers, some less tangible and more cultural issues are listed. These include lack of training and knowledge, gender stereotyping of activities, planning issues, competition from other subjects, colleagues undervaluing PE, and other attitude complaints.

At the risk of sounding naive, we see and hear the same concerns in the medical profession. Young teachers, like young doctors, generally start with an enormous capacity for care and empathy. The grind of the job can wear a person down and allow us to lose sight of why we chose our professions. Our jobs in medicine and education should start in an amazingly simple place: We want to create an atmosphere that allows people to be honest and comfortable with who they are. We need to express—and I say this not for the want of a better word— love for our patients and students. Children especially will respond to this—particularly children who have never felt the concern and love from an adult for simply being their true selves. This acceptance can be a powerful place to begin to remove the roadblocks to change.

Unfortunately, the student-related barriers ghost many of the teacher-related barriers in that attitude and psychology are paramount. Lack of student engagement, not liking the activities, lack of motivation, sedentary behavior, peer pressure, lack of peer support, and socioeconomic issues all make the list. It would seem for such important problems there should be aggressive work toward solutions, but with myriad other issues confronted by school staff on a daily basis, these roadblocks do not seem to get the attention they might deserve. It breaks my heart, but this generation has lost its physical identity and might be beyond saving.

A classroom teacher responds:

> If educators are opposed to adequate physical education in schools, it is likely without understanding the benefits of physical activity on students' health and learning. Pressure to perform (and to get students to perform) may be a leading reason classroom teachers ignore these benefits and become greedy about their time with students. After all, they are responsible for preparing students for standardized tests used to hold schools and teachers accountable.
>
> At our K–8 school, space and time dictate the number of PE classes we can even offer in 1 week. With nine grade levels and only one gymnasium in a town with long winters keeping students indoors, we max out the opportunities to use our gym and still leave most students with fewer than 2 hours each week spent in PE class.

3: What Are PE Teachers Being Taught?

What started out as "normal" schools to educate teachers are now hundreds of colleges and universities across the country. The number of degrees granted in PE, however, seems to have peaked, and there are now fewer being granted than in the past, no doubt reflecting the decreased emphasis on PE in schools. In this section, we will take a brief look at what a PE student coming out of college has been studying, using the example of Springfield College in Massachusetts, which has a history of excellence in teacher education.

Springfield College began granting degrees for PE majors in 1887 and claims the inventors of basketball and volleyball on its list of alumni. Prospective PE teachers "complete the movement and sports studies major, related physical education courses, and an extensive practicum component." Students start with "general education" classes with an aim toward "educating the whole person in spirit, mind, and body for leadership in service to humanity." The list of "core requirements" reads like the lists of topics in some of the state standards. Over 4 years, the student will take classes in physiology, kinesiology, anatomy, math, motor learning, physics of movement, coaching, outdoor education, leadership, and psychology of sport, among others. Physical education teacher programs appear to be moving from a sports and skills-centered model to a more comprehensive movement and health-centered model. This change should help PE teachers advance the cause of overall public health, but we cannot lose sight of the main goal for children in PE classes: They need to be moving!

Though most PE teachers are well educated, one problem is that these professionals are not always the ones doing the teaching. Many school districts allow classroom teachers and others to teach PE. Indeed, 68% of elementary schools allow classroom teachers to teach physical education. Certification of middle/junior high school and high school physical education teachers is required in only 82% and 90% of states respectively (NASPE). Also, many of the PE teachers are overwhelmed with the number of students and the limited time they have for instruction. Graduates of Springfield College and similar institutions are coming out with the knowledge needed to help our students with a life of activity. They have the tools to follow the various standards (which of course were usually written by physical educators!). We need to give them the support, the funds, and importantly, the *time* to use their education for the benefit of our youth.

John Cawley with the National Bureau of Economic Research did an interesting study back in 2005, looking at some of these incredibly important issues (2005). He found students were only getting *16 minutes* of activity per class and felt that PE time had "no detectable impact on youth body mass index (BMI)." His data was collected just after the enactment of No Child Left Behind, and he notes the percentage of high school PE dropped from 42% in 1991 to 28% in 2003, and *daily* PE dropped in middle school from 17% to 6% in that time. Sadly, this dearth of PE did not motivate the students to rush out after school to burn some energy—just the opposite. His data also shows 26% of schools nationally did not comply with state standards (consistent with my own survey results), feeling this "implies that schools may not respond to tougher state standards." He admits in his study that P.E. classes have been criticized for taking a "roll out the balls and let them play approach, in which there is no organized activity and no assurance that each student is physically active." The one questionably optimistic finding was that children participating in sports generally had lower BMIs, but this was titrated to how many sports they were playing. Students who played three sports had lower BMIs than those only participating in one. As we will see in the next chapter, only 16% of students in my survey were three-sport athletes

Cawley acknowledges he did not study the "quality" of the PE. As most of us know, if a teacher is unmotivated, the students will follow suit. I blame my loss of interest in math to my sophomore-year teacher in high school. There is no excuse for this in PE as most children are keen to play due to the primitive aspects of their brain wiring. Punishing children by taking away gym or recess time is just the opposite of what they need for discipline or academics. Regarding time, again, that can be the fault of the teachers but more so, the system. Just like in an operating room, every teacher needs to maximize every minute they have with their students. The fact that some PE teachers are "physical identity killers" by not keeping these youngsters moving emphasizes the need for oversight by the principals or better, the PE czar.

There has been occasional talk of a federal mandate to establish compulsory PE across the country. This reminds me of the motto of Rene Dubos, asking us to "think globally, but act locally" (Sack, 2018). I believe this is ultimately a local issue as long as we listen to the global research. We know the global recommendations and knowledge; we must bring these now to the community level, to every school in every school district, accepting administrative help from the federal and state governments.

4: Are We "Waist Deep in the Big Muddy?"

This old Pete Seeger song might be a perfect metaphor for where we are with the state of PE in America. I never met Mr. Seeger but feel as if I knew him, having lived part of my life upriver from his home in the Hudson Valley. The song, based on a true story, describes following someone into a swamp who refuses to change course, despite the rising water. I am not pessimistic by nature; however, at some point, you need to look at the research, put your previous thoughts, prejudices, and perhaps your "experience" to the side, and chart a new course.

Similar to other public health issues, children's future well-being is truly at risk unless we make a cultural change: a PE revolution. In this case, we actually know what the problems are: sedentary behavior coupled with bad food producing obesity, depression, boredom, and a loss of physical identity. Declining time for PE class periods is the first and easiest problem to tackle and can be done immediately, at absolutely no cost. We know this is not only good physically for the students, but good academically (Rasberry et al., 2011). President Kennedy elucidated the aspirations and ways forward for our country's health. Yet 50 years later, with all of our knowledge and understanding of the obesity crisis, we still have not found our way. We have all heard the definition of insanity linked to Albert Einstein (though apparently it's a misattribution) as "doing the same thing over and over again and expecting different results." No matter who it is ascribed to, we have, as a nation, repeated our mistakes regarding fitness on many fronts. On some level, I suspect we could blame this useless repetition on our primitive brain, as we know it can sometimes work against us. Nevertheless, in the realm of physical education and fitness, we are at a crossroads, and it is time to let our cognitive brain reasoning take the helm.

CHAPTER 4

Removing the Roadblocks
Establishing Rebranded Physical Education

MOTHER NATURE'S LAST STAND

I am not a pessimist by nature. As a doctor, I know that showing patience and allowing Mother Nature to work is often all that is needed for healing. That said, we know in these early stages of the new century, things are distinctly *not* moving in a healing direction for our children's health—just the contrary. Every time you open a newspaper, it seems there is an article describing a decline in overall fitness, coupled with an increase in "diseases of civilization" or "Western diseases" such as obesity, heart disease, high blood pressure, type 2 diabetes, and osteoporosis (Carrera-Bastos et al., 2010). Doctors are often blamed for treating illness and injuries once they happen when we should be focused on prevention and well-being. Part of my job as a physician is to ask: What am I doing today for my patients' health in the future?

My belief in the past was that if we model appropriate behavior for our children by getting outside as a family, having fresh vegetables at communal meals, limiting screen time, and so on, they will internalize such behaviors. Although our children might go through phases of rebellion with bad food choices, too much time spent on video games, and perhaps even vaping, their primitive brains should eventually kick in and right the "healthy living" ship. But this is not the case, and there is evidence that their questionable choices are actually changing brain chemistry, making it that much harder to achieve a healthy lifestyle. Mother Nature is losing this battle, and we are running out of time for a change in tactics to avoid losing the war. The poisons of today—the scientifically tested ultra-processed foods with their combinations of salt, sugar, and fat; the equally scientifically tested video games and social media; and an overall sedentary lifestyle are having the same health effects as cigarettes did two generations ago. Children actually become addicted on many levels to these new vices (Aliyari, 2015; Park et al., 2017; Pujol et al., 2016). Young people are *not* eventually losing interest in these terrible choices. The pendulum is *not* swinging back to the things many of us find "natural" such as a bike ride, fresh fruit, or playing in the park. We have been waiting for Mother Nature to heal things for the past five decades. This health crisis is the human equivalent of climate change. The good news is that we know what we need to do, and it will cost far less than any environmental legislation.

In the previous chapter we reviewed some of the national and state literature describing an efficient PE program and how there seems to be little disagreement among experts regarding children's need for exercise both physically and cognitively. Where the disagreement comes is how to go about making change happen on the local level, what specifically those changes might look like, and oh yeah, how to pay for them.

My criteria for school PE are simple:

- It must be daily.
- It must increase the heart rate.
- It must be egalitarian.
- It must be fun!

With these criteria in place, PE will promote *physical identity,* which will support physical, emotional, and academic health, the ultimate goal of the entire enterprise. These criteria are not created from whimsy. They are based on the best available science, experience, and data.

MONEY, MONEY EVERYWHERE, BUT NOT A DROP FOR PE

A man in my town was a great one for writing to the local newspaper complaining about absolutely any increase in taxes, including those going to the school budget. His argument was always the same: First, we can't afford it. Second, we don't need it. Third, there is no proof that throwing money at something is going to help the situation. Everyone knew Mert (and I suspect he has a doppelgänger in your town), and though he died years ago, his name is still invoked when discussing any town expenditure. Although Mert and I had friendly clashes in

sharper scheduling pencil. PE must stop being thought of as a luxury item that only rich districts can afford. We need to make changes so the system can work for every child, in every community. What we absolutely do *not* need is to lessen PE. We need urgency and intention to make PE daily and better. There is no STEM without FITNESS.

Without enforcing standards, the time, money, and energy will never be found for PE. It is not the fault of the PE teachers, as they will not change their ways unless driven to do so. This is simply human nature; the primitive brain in this case is working against us. I spoke of how the medical profession has begun to adopt evidence-based standards. Another big shift for the medical community was a majority of doctors switching from private practice to become hospital employees. Hospital rules included being forced to move from written charts to electronic medical records (EMR). It was a huge change in culture, but it was mandated by the hospitals, who were often taking their orders from government agencies and insurance companies. Similar to student math scores, money from the federal government was used as an incentive for using EMR, and the hospitals were now signing the doctors' paychecks. So guess what? Doctors, the most elitist, obstinate, and obsessive group of people that exist, changed their behavior. My belief is that if we can turn around a group like doctors, whose culture prescribed bleeding as a medical treatment for centuries, we should be able to turn the tide on today's culture of PE.

Money issues aside, many people, whether administrators, teachers, or the public, are against change on "principle," though when probed they have a difficult time explaining how they developed such principles. In fact, attempts at cultural change are not new and are happening all the time, in multiple forms. There were successful national campaigns against smoking, littering, and drunk driving, but there are also similar influences at every level of government. In New Hampshire, signs entering the state read "Drive courteously. It's the New Hampshire way!" On a more local level, when I was a student in Stony Brook, New York, the trash cans had printed on them a quote attributed to Abe Lincoln that said, "I like to see a man proud of the place in which he lives." Are these examples of indoctrination or simply nudging people toward behavior for the greater good? I am not calling for presidents, governors, school administrators, or even teachers to replace family and philosophic beliefs as the moral compass for our students. I am asking all parties to take the concept of physical identity to heart and create an educational atmosphere of fun and health for all children.

A classroom teacher responds:

A before-school jump rope club energizes and grounds students for seemingly a good part of the morning. I can assure you that this simple approach is of great benefit to all participants. Call it a gathering of friends. Call it a chance to have older students mentor younger, less experienced students. Call it a call to arms in which students come to recognize that fitness through play is worthwhile. Just know that this seemingly simple adjustment to school life can have a profound effect.

IF YOU CAN'T TEACH, DON'T TEACH PE: GOAL SETTING FOR THE 21ST CENTURY PE TEACHER

Okay—it must be said sometime, so let's get it out of the way. Remember the old saying, "if you can't do, teach; if you can't teach, teach PE"? Well I am here to tell you that nothing could be further from the truth in this rebranded PE. In fact, *the PE teacher needs to be the lynchpin for learning in the school.* Let me explain.

Malcolm Gladwell talks in his book *The Tipping Point* about Paul Revere being a "connector" in Boston society (2014). Revere knew a lot of people and a lot about what was going on. He was the one you wanted to meet in the pub after being away for a few months. *PE teachers should be the great connector in schools.* They need to know what all the students are doing, learning, struggling with, who is causing trouble, when the British are coming (just checking to see if you are still paying attention!), generally every nuance about what could be limiting academic and personal success. These ideas put a lot on PE teachers—but they have the training and the knowledge. They know what they should be doing and what they *can* be doing. This is where a PE assistant would be helpful—and justified. Sadly, almost all the PE teachers I have spoken with feel limited by the "system" and the old ways of thinking. We need to give PE professionals the tools we know are important for success from the last chapter: leadership training, more time with students, consults with other teachers, help from the czar, respect from the principals, and so on, to help us pull us out of this health crisis.

A PE teacher responds:

It is no secret that gym teachers have historically been marginalized in our schools. I periodically despair that trying to alter such attitudes is a losing battle. I want to be an agent for positive change but . . .

As has been stated in no uncertain terms, fit students make better learners (Fedewa, 2011). Trained PE teachers should be spending their time designing and supervising multiple grade-level programs and be available to guide students through any rough times. If a child is struggling in a particular subject, the classroom teacher and PE teacher can work together on a strategy. This is why the PE assistants are so vital. The PE assistant frees the PE teacher's schedule to create that environment of caring, comfort and, hopefully, excitement, to find the full potential and physical identity in every student. These are not new concepts, but they are increasingly lost in our fast-paced, computer-driven world, particularly in the fields of education and medicine. Students, like patients in a doctor's office, need measures of time, quiet, and focus just on them. They need to know that someone cares, that someone understands their individual needs, even if just for a few moments. This is something that cannot only shape the life of the student or patient but can be equally satisfying for the teacher and doctor.

Here's an example: "James" is 12 years old and at the beginning of the school year is struggling to get his homework completed. He does poorly on the first tests. The classroom teacher has discussed this with him, but there has not been any improvement. The PE teacher could then be consulted. This is potentially a person who knows James from the previous year(s), and with the relationship alluded to above, has established a level of trust. He or she would discuss—on a more adult level now that he is in middle school—some of the roadblocks that are getting in the way of him completing his assignments. This might involve a changed family situation affecting his life at home, his sleep, his nutrition, and of course, his activity. James is on the edge of puberty and is not regarded by his peers as an athlete. His outdoor play is becoming less, and his video play more. This is a student who is struggling and needs some one-on-one help. "Hungry listening" followed by some loving guidance can make a huge difference when coming from an adult the student knows and trusts. Although no one wants to be singled out, it is done in other subjects and can be similarly done effectively with PE. This is why it is vital the administration treat the PE folks similarly to their colleagues in the classroom: We want them to never forget they are teachers, and they should be acting as such. James and the PE teacher would come up with some *strategies* of how they can work exercise into his schedule, *ideally before his toughest classes.* At the same time the possibility of coming into school early for exercise and getting breakfast (tragically, this is needed and thus offered more and more [School Breakfast Program, n.d.]), and after-school exercise suggestions *before* doing his homework and playing his video games (ideally quantifying his screen time knowing we cannot stop it completely). In this manner the PE teacher is not in the same category as the "nagging" (sorry but . . .) classroom teacher or parent, but an ally and partner. It is this planning and attention to detail that should be the role of the PE teacher. The PE assistant meanwhile is running a class or supervising students doing their individualized programs.

I use the word "strategy" often in my sports medicine and sport psychology practices. This word is often worked in with the phrase, "I just make suggestions. I am not telling you how to live your life." Our fictional James (and there are dozens of Jameses in every school) is at the age where he wants more freedom and needs his voice to be heard. As we discussed earlier, PE is a great place for this. With the teacher *and* the student coming up with a *strategy,* it feels less like a set of rules but suggestions to make his or her life *easier.* This is terribly important for them to understand. Convincing the students it is simply easier to do the (even minimal amount of) work, to pass the tests, to be efficient with time, will have positive effects on their lives for years to come.

Not only should it be the responsibility of the PE teacher to help the classroom teacher, but it is also their job to help the music and art teachers get activity into their classes. A game of "musical chairs" could be more of a learning experience if, rather than sitting when the music stops, the students could sit with an octave or timing change. Also, the child that gets left out would continue to move and help "coach" another player. Every participant is listening to the music and still moving because *we're in motion.* Marching band and chorus with dance moves, art that has the students getting outside with their paints or cameras—the options are endless with just a bit of thought. The children are in motion, they are learning, and they are doing. All teachers should be aware of the data. PE might be the subject that has the strongest influence on the health and success of the child as they advance in school. Yes, you can have a huge influence teaching chemistry, but I would contend not as easily and not affecting as many students in the long run as teaching PE.

An administrator replies:

> One thing that stood out to me was "physical education must stop being thought of as a luxury item that only rich school districts can afford." I have never thought of it that way and not sure I agree. We are lucky in our schools that it is a requirement vs. some other districts. Perhaps requiring P.E. each year with some growth goals would be something we could support as an administrative team. The time issue though . . .

CONTAGIONS YOU WANT TO CATCH

It would not be effective to enact the rebranded PE revolution piece-meal. Nibbling around the edges would not show the hoped for physical and academic improvements and will give the naysayers reason to scuttle any changes. As I will emphasize again and again, it does not take more money; it takes leadership and will. Human nature makes it difficult for anyone in a small community such as a school to directly criticize others. Though teacher discipline is generally the charge of the principal, it is a delicate balance that many people are simply not comfortable with. This is where the czars should help, as there needs to be some level of enforcement. It is the role of the czar or his or her (volunteer) assistants to observe classes, look at lesson plans, help procure needed equipment or funds, and convince the local teacher to enact appropriate change. Much of this could even be done online with the local schools submitting videos of their classes. If using video, have the camera focus on the students who are not normally predisposed to athletics. Are these children having fun? Do they have a smile on their faces? These are the students we want to see in motion.

A contest they have every year in Ireland is called "Tidy Towns." This is an all-volunteer, community effort with prizes given out in multiple categories for, you guessed it, the tidiest town. Winners are announced in all the papers and other media outlets. The contest has become hugely popular and a source of bragging rights across the country. Signs proudly noting they were Tidy Town winners remain for years. This is an example of a "social contagion" with the only incentive being satisfaction and pride.

We have these incentives for school sports teams but imagine if we could establish sought after prizes for PE *programs*. Imagine if each state governor recognized the importance of *overall* student fitness, taking a page out of the early PSAL in New York City where overall participation counted? The PE teacher could then garner support not only at the state level, but also from local sports medicine doctors, coaches, dance instructors, chiropractors, yogis, and more, all helping make the program a success. These folks could also up the ante, asking for support from the czar and state government for other community resources such as exercise trails, bike lanes, playgrounds, and the like. The interest is there; it just needs to be organized and harnessed.

COMPETITIVE SPORTS ARE SPORTS—THEY ARE RARELY PE

As we wind down the discussion of roadblocks for proper PE, we are forced to again consider one of the most controversial topics: Sports vs. PE. Competitive sports established an "education" position over the years, with no data to support such prestige (Hyman, 2012). Furthermore, some sports have taken on more value than others in the school landscape, particularly football. By this time, I think you know where I come down in this debate. Young people today need active play and exercise first, *then* sports.

Let me be clear: *I have no problem with sports as long as they do not push out play and PE.* The sports model has been waxing and waning in the realm of PE for over 100 years, but varsity sports have not always existed in the role they currently serve. We saw how Holderness School, an institution with a strong physical identity, uses sports exclusively for physical activity. Unfortunately, as I tell the young ski racers who try to emulate local New Hampshire hero Bode Miller by adopting some of his less traditional techniques, "you are probably not Bode." Using a sports model that successfully translates into fitness for all is rare. As a result, unless the only students at your school are the ones who chose to go there, as at Holderness, schools should consider a model that ensures everyone is physically involved, not just the motivated few. Parenthetically, Bode is not just a great skier, but excels in many sports including tennis and soccer.

Although in a perfect world the sports model can help children learn skills and hopefully have fun, it simply does not work in the limited time dedicated to PE. Many players will not be participating at an aggressive level as they do not have the background or motivation to develop such skills, and this is particularly true for girls. Baseball and softball, while prototypical American sports, are perfect examples of activities that need too much skill to be used as exercise for the vast majority of participants. In the limited time for PE, most sports will not have *all the students* achieving the physiological response of increased heart rate, muscle loading, and other desired calorie-burning and endorphin-producing responses. The PE teacher would have to work impossibly hard to ensure all students get their needed exercise from just doing sports activities. The importance of aggressive physical exercise is even more vital for the children who might have special needs, such as those who struggle with attention-deficit/hyperactivity disorder (ADHD). In a study from Italy children with ADHD were put on either a program of endurance types of exercise (e.g., walking, skipping, some manner of constant motion) vs. more standard PE of drills with a ball. The children who kept moving with endurance-type exercise showed the most improvement on subsequent attention testing (Reynolds, 2011). Ideally, we can have both, and we give examples of this in Chapter 5. Ultimately, the primary goals should be burning calories, improving cognition, and maintaining physical identity.

LIFELONG ACTIVITIES

I am all in on sports *in addition to* PE, especially if they can be considered lifelong activities. Many water, snow, and basic ball sports would be in this category. One of the analogies I give when deciding what constitutes a lifelong activity is, oddly enough, the Olympics. (I am about to make more enemies—but here goes.) In my opinion, to qualify as an Olympic sport, the first criterion is that you must know who won *the instant the event is over*. Track events—obvious Olympic sports. A gymnastics event—not so much. If we are waiting for "judges" to tell us who wins, it might be a perfectly good sport, but it should not be an Olympic sport. One of the sports I covered at the professional level was ski jumping. It never made sense to me that they awarded "style points" when there is a perfectly easy way to tell who wins—the person who jumped the furthest!

Similarly, we need to be discriminating regarding any sports associated with school PE. Tennis and golf are great sports and potential lifelong activities, but as ball and stick sports they do not qualify. Few people play sports such as baseball or football after the age of 18. They take skills most people do not possess (such as hitting a ball or enjoying being tackled). In addition, they require a big field and a lot of expensive equipment. Maybe worst of all, the children playing these sports are standing around too much. Baseball and football and others are excellent community sports, but they are not great sports to burn calories, engage multiple muscle qualities, and allow participation of all students. Public school PE needs to be for average students (thus excluding children in Lake Wobegon) and, I would argue, students who struggle to achieve. Any extra dollars in the school budget for sports should go to programs that emphasize fitness for life and meet our criteria of constant motion and elevated heart rate: cycling, skiing, surfing, kayaking, dance, and so on. Taxpayer money is limited. Ensuring lifelong physical identity is time sensitive. *Most present-day school sports do not make the cut to be part of the rebranded PE or even as school lifelong activity programs.* Sorry. But by my criteria most of these sports can be in the Olympics, if that helps.

For lifelong sports, there are many well-researched, evidence-based models and programs for the modern PE teacher to discover. Examples of programs and philosophies that fit the criteria for fun and fitness are the Coordinated Approach to Child Health (CATCH), PE4life, and Sports, Play, and Active Recreation for Kids (SPARK) (Melanie & Carrie,1970; About SPARK, n.d.). With lifelong activities, while I tend to think of winter sports because of where I live, teachers in southern regions could introduce kayaking, swimming, canoeing, paddle boarding, surfing, in-line skating, and mountain biking. Those in cities could organize cycling, running, skateboarding, dance, yoga, jump rope, and ultimate frisbee games. Planning for these activities are labor intensive; thus the czars and their local connections should prove especially useful.

I was involved with our local middle school ski program that had stopped for several years due to lack of leadership. It took a couple of teachers to get this wonderful school activity off life support. One positive of our Internet world is once these programs are organized with information and contacts established, they can almost run themselves with a few annual emails. It would break my heart if every child in the mountains of Colorado was not introduced to skiing, just as it would be a crime if someone on the coast of Florida did not feel comfortable in the ocean or anyone, anywhere, could not ride a bike. These would all fit the category of being lifelong activities.

At this point I suspect my sport psychologist wishes are taking over my interests as a taxpayer. I have said throughout that the program I propose will be cost neutral. When words like skiing and surfing are bandied about, I can almost see hands shooting into the air. Yes, the activities I describe take some organizing and perhaps extra funding, but they can be the grist for a superior education and engaged students. This is where the czar, local professional sports teams, community groups such as the YMCA, Boys and Girls Clubs, and simply individuals with an interest in giving back come into play. Is there a yoga instructor willing to donate some time, a running club, a pool or beach nearby? Yes, it will take some energy, but this is the stuff of a "village." With these lifelong sports activities, the interest, caring, and enthusiasm of the teachers and other adults are displayed outside the school. These activities can also serve as a proud connection to their neighborhood and hometown: a place we hope the students will settle and raise their own families. They need to be shown and learn to appreciate this world, their world.

IF EXERGAMING IS MY ONLY OPTION, GIVE ME FOOTBALL

In this final segment regarding roadblocks for the new PE, we will touch on a subject I am completely incapable of discussing with any objectivity (yes—up to now this entire book has been free of bias): that being the use (or misuse) of screen time in PE. As we all know, it is the rare child over the age of 12 who does not have a smartphone in his or her pocket (or ear!) as well as some type of gaming console at home. Using applications for these devices, a new word has emerged: "exergaming." Exergaming basically uses technologies such as video or virtual reality and requires participants to be physically active while they play (What Is Exergaming?). Perhaps not surprising at this relatively early stage, data for the efficacy of exergaming is lacking (Faric et al., 2019; Fu et al., 2019). Also, perhaps not surprisingly, I am not in favor of these products, as they do not engage our primitive brain, but a brain that is being altered by two-dimensional screen exposure, precisely what we are trying to decrease in our children's lives. As exergames do not get the player outside in the fresh air, they will be dubiously useful for feeding our physical identity as they are not exposing the person to the most intense input imaginable: Mother Nature.

I understand the concept of exergames: Anything that can get somebody moving, even a little, is a plus. I would propose that this is another example of being told that the old presentation (i.e., the natural world) is just not interesting enough for young people today. This can be a self-fulfilling prophecy. Nature, even in a city, has enough wonder and interest that it does not have to be supplemented by technology. If we continue to stimulate ourselves above the primitive brain level, we become numb. No doubt the tech manufacturers are happy to present their products, most of which are part of the problem, as part of the solution (at a significant price!). If our biophilia and physical identity is not muted early, it will not diminish, but increase with time, and exergaming would cease to be a "thing."

For similar reasons, I cannot strongly support any online learning when it comes to PE. The fact that some schools allow students to fulfill their PE requirements online is anathema to everything I believe and what my physical identity longs for. Learning about your body, your fitness, and your health is always a good thing. Allowing this to represent the same thing as burning calories running is ridiculous. The only time this would be reasonable is if a student was *truly* medically unable to play. These students could spend the time reading PE-related subjects. For a young child, this might mean reading a well-written biography of an athlete or soldier (e.g., JFK, Wilma Rudolph, Muhammad Ali), or for the older students, perhaps a book on sport psychology, sport sociology, or sports medicine (see how I did that?).

Presented to this point is a view of what PE can and should look like on the local level. In this rebranded or, as they say in Illinois, "enhanced" PE, I suggest full use of the state PE czar and the PE teacher's assistants. These folks are key from either side of the equation, as the PE teacher has a different role in the rebranded PE than in the past. I am not naive, but like René Dubos, I am a "despairing optimist" (1977). I sincerely believe we as a culture can do this. There is sound science to back up the change to this type of program. Such positive change will not be possible, however, unless we make some difficult funding decisions. Let's start tackling the money question, since as we all know, when they say it's not about the money . . .

"THERE'S NO TELLING WHERE THE MONEY WENT"

As the grandson of Irish immigrants and the son of a child raised during the Great Depression, frugality never needed to be explained to me. And a frugal childhood was just the beginning. My chemistry professor felt that for undergrads, good science only needed a bench, some glassware, a few items in the stockroom, and imagination. I was thus well prepared for a state-funded, unendowed medical school that eventually led to starting a practice as the first orthopedic surgeon in a small town in northern New Hampshire. At each stop money was limited, but it was never a significant roadblock to progress.

Many opportunities for betterment, including changes in the behemoths of education and health care, are often lost due to financial concerns. One difference is we now appreciate that education and health care are connected well beyond the school nurse. As we have discussed, physical health and fitness are intimately connected to learning. Unfortunately, our children are increasingly being pressured by a super-aggressive media and an unwitting school system to make poor health decisions. More directed advertising of questionable products, more unhealthy food options in the cafeteria and vending machines, more social pressure to make bad choices, more time indoors and sadly, *less* time and funding for outdoor fun and physical education. Teachers and parents are almost powerless against the work of the professional marketers who spend their lives learning how to influence our children at every turn. And though teachers and parents are *not* powerless at our local schools, they have abdicated their influence when it comes to the vital subject of physical education. Whenever anyone brings up the topic of a change in any aspect of school, PE or otherwise, someone in the room (usually Mert) will shout, "We can't afford it." The words "increase in budget" have not yet been uttered— everyone just assumes they will be in the next sentence.

It frustrates me when governments seem to always find money for various pet projects, but then claim belts tightened to their maximum level when it comes to spending for education or health care. This does not mean I am in favor of giving bureaucrats and government officials the codes to my bank account. I would not last another day in the Granite State with an attitude like that! Also, I am not foolish enough to wade into a debate of what spending is necessary and what is expendable (that I save for the pub). I *am* foolish enough to say that as taxpayers, few of us have any clue who is paying their share, where our tax dollars go, and how those dollars are spent. At the end of the day, there really *is* no telling where the money went. Trying to figure out where our tax dollars go has stumped some of the best forensic accountants, as the paths of money circulating through the federal, state, and local governments are Byzantine at best. Like most everyone, I become incensed when I hear about government waste, politicians on the take, or citizens cheating the system (all too common in medicine especially with Medicare and disability payments). But that's lost money—I can't even follow the money we know exists. For example, the fate of one pot of money particularly bothers me, as we are told that by supporting it we are helping our children's education. That pot is the lottery.

The lottery might be the poster child of "there's no telling where the money went." Theoretically, lottery money in many states, including my own, is said to go to "education." However, most data show that when money does run to education, it is not a net plus, as this lottery money simply substitutes for previously dedicated money (Henricks & Embrick, 2017). No school administrator has ever told me they had more money to spend one year because more people bought lottery tickets. The lottery (and now sports betting) arguably results in a regressive tax that finds its way into state coffers, not to your local schools (Goldman, 2014).

As taxpayers, it is our job to elect representatives who have the best interests of the community's citizens at heart while keeping track of our money. We then need to educate these officials where the money would most effectively be spent. I would submit a great place to start investing these tax dollars is toward our increasingly unhealthy children, as they will be responsible for our own health needs in the near future. And the way to make these students less unhealthy is through physical education at school. And, by the way, we actually do have the money.

FOLLOW THE MONEY

When planning this section, I hoped to "follow the money" for multiple high school athletic and physical education budgets. In this age of the Internet, I thought it would be a slam dunk. The first budget I looked at was a high school of just under 1,000 students in the Northeast. Their proposed budget gave line-by-line numbers for the various sports as well as other expenses. "This is fantastic," I thought, "as I can easily collect data to make my case for improved PE programs." Additionally, because I cited Massachusetts, California, Mississippi, New Hampshire, and Illinois when discussing state standards, I thought I would do a "deeper dive" into these states, comparing multiple schools. It might turn into a mind-numbing exercise, but it would allow clear comparisons.

Then, as they say, the wheels fell off.

As a start, it turned out at the time of this bit of research (2017) that many schools in Illinois were not proposing budgets due to the fact that the State of Illinois had not passed their own spending plan, leaving the schools, all of whom depend heavily on state funding, in limbo. (It surprised me how much vitriol was aimed at the Illinois governor himself on the school district websites!) The other block in Illinois was trying to tease out the schools in Chicago as they were folded into the full city education budget.

Moving on from Illinois, things did not get easier. Similar to the district-by-district differences in physical education programs, there was no commonality in reporting of "where the money went." The posting of school budgets was as individual as the schools themselves. Some districts provided a plethora of information, while others bore witness to a spartan model of accounting. And alas, some schools had essentially no information posted, and I suspect one would have to attend the school board meetings or go to the town hall to examine any written reports. Some documents broke the athletic budget out of the full school budget, while others had it buried in a maze of other numbers.

One of my favorite (?!?!) school budgets came from the Midwest. This is a large, suburban school district, the kind I imagine would be the envy of most of the country. That said, they did not make understanding their budget easy. The district would be considered relatively well to do with only 28% of the kids obtaining free and reduced lunch (see definition below). Their budget document runs a full 469 pages with athletic expenditures embedded throughout. The student "activity fund (entertainment, publications . . . extra-curricular activities . . .")" is 1.2% of the entire budget. They are said to spend $18 million for building and grounds, an incredible 9% of the entire budget, and $6.5 million for transportation, some 3.4% of the budget. Notably in my reading of this document, I just could not tell what percentage of these numbers were specifically for sports or PE. And that's the problem.

Here are some of the sports-related line items in their yearly budget:

- "out of district travel–touchdown" = $2,291
- "purchased services–soccer boys" = $282
- "purchased services–touchdown club" = $15,934

- "supplies" for cheerleaders = $48,872
- "supplies" for baseball = $9,809
- "supplies" for football club = $36,323
- "supplies" for volleyball = $22,843
- "purchased services" for football = $20,682
- "purchased services" for wrestling = $11,149

For the other high school in the district these were some of the line items:

- "purchased services" football = $13,282
- "football equipment" = $14,194
- "purchased services" boys golf = $14,844
- "purchased services" girls golf = $3,828

The problem with trying to understand this enormous document is that athletic spending is in so many places it is difficult to get a clear picture of "where the money went." If we just used the two line items for "athletics and intramurals" for the two high schools, it would be only 0.3% of the district budget, one of the smallest numbers I calculated from my national search. And no, I have no idea what "purchased services" entails or the differences between "football," the "football club," and the "touchdown club." But at least there are numbers documented so a taxpayer in this school district might be able to question them, if that is any consolation.

Eventually, I enlisted the services of a trained accountant to help navigate through the budget mazes, but most often the numbers were just not available. By pointing all this out, I do not mean to indicate subterfuge or poor stewardship. I have no doubt most school financial administrators are honest, typically overworked civil servants. What these budget records support, however, is my Robert Palmer theory of taxes: We have a general ignorance of where the money is coming from, and then how, where, and on what, it is spent.

Despite a life in the medical business, if you asked me, or almost any doctor for that matter, to break down your medical bills, it would be a Sisyphean task. Certainly, in my searches for the school athletic budgets I would often come to a roadblock, some of which I was able to get around, but often feeling like it was being made deliberately difficult. One school district wanted me to get a password to look at the budget—and contact the school to do so! Whenever I see announcements that certain school board meetings are not open to the public, I become uneasy. I appreciate these boards cannot function if being constantly interrupted by what some might consider minutiae. Perhaps in an effort toward full disclosure, they might broadcast the proceedings so interested viewers could submit their concerns by post or email. At the end of the day, it is the taxpayers' money, and they should have a clear idea how it is being spent.

If things are not lucid for me working with an accountant, they are probably not lucid for most citizens. Here's another great example: one southern city's school budget is some $141 million, but no clear accounting for athletic spending. The only line item I could find in this 185-page document was categorized under "fixed formulas/amounts," and under "athletics" they noted a high school student would be calculated to cost $14,850, though it is not obvious where that precise number comes from or what it is for. This compared to a middle school student figure of $10,000 and elementary of $0! ROTC students were given a yearly expenditure of $3,000, though again, it is not at all clear what this money is funding, why it is a city expenditure and not federal, and so on. My accountant consultant, someone who spent many years in city government, was equally baffled.

With this in mind, I felt a change in strategy was needed, so I decided to contact school athletic directors (ADs) directly. As my main interest was spending on sports as compared to PE, I narrowed my search to only high school ADs. Like my office survey of why parents involved their children in organized sports, this was not constructed to be a scientific analysis of data. It would, however, give us information by not counting on what may or may not have been recorded in the published school budgets, but access data directly from the people who are running the programs. Thus, in the following pages I will present survey data from multiple schools in the 2017–2018 school year in an attempt to present a qualitative snapshot of a number of issues regarding school sports and PE. A truly quantitative investigation is almost impossible unless one has complete access to all the school's accounting and athletic program records for the past number of years.

IF YOU WANT TO KNOW SOMETHING, MAYBE JUST ASK

Several years ago, I was on the board of directors of a local health care service that provides physical therapy, visiting nurses, and hospice care.

This was a great organization that took wonderful care of many of my patients. Though I had never previously served on a board, when asked I was more than happy to do so—at least for the first 5 minutes. I should have known from my 2-week stint as chief of surgery (that was not a typo—it might have been less than 2 weeks—I know I presided over only exactly one staff meeting) that I am genetically incapable of serving in such a role. I hate sitting, I hate enclosed rooms, I hate Robert's Rules of Order, I hate lukewarm coffee, and I hate shuffling papers. The final straw was our board chair suggesting we all take a course on how to read a spreadsheet. After serving my term, I was mercifully not asked to stay. All of this to say, athletic directors (ADs) have different strengths and weaknesses. Some are interested in the details of the business side, though for most this is the worst aspect of the job. Thus, out of respect for like-minded souls, I purposely asked the ADs for broad strokes when answering my questions. To get a quantitative tally of all the expenses—from personnel to facilities to transportation to officiating to equipment to depreciation, and so on, would be well past most ADs' patience for some doctor from New Hampshire. I assured the athletic directors their schools would not be identified individually, only by state.

These were my questions:

1. Where is your school located?
2. What is the enrollment for grades 9–12?
3. How many PE teachers are on staff for grades 9–12?
4. What is the average salary of a full-time PE teacher?
5. Over the course of 4 years, how much PE are students required to take (minutes per week)?
6. Does PE time differ from grades 9 through 12?
7. Are your PE requirements based on state standards?
8. What percent of your high school students play a varsity sport?
9. What percent of your high school students play three varsity sports (i.e., are participating the entire school year)?
10. What percent of your sports coaches are not teachers on staff?
11. What is the annual budget for sports/athletics?
12. What is the annual budget for physical education?

There were many other questions I would like to have asked the ADs, but getting such information in a cold survey is not easy to obtain from these busy individuals, even with the offered $10 honorarium. The questions I did ask were for these reasons:

- The location question is obvious. As hoped, we had respondents from across the country thus giving a reasonable snapshot for the entire nation.
- The enrollment and number of PE teachers allowed me to calculate this ratio. It is my contention that offering multiple organized sports presents a greater disadvantage to small schools and schools from poorer socioeconomic areas. This is because fielding 20+ varsity teams (a common number in many school districts) will represent a larger percentage of a small school's overall budget. If money is being spent on sports, this means potentially less money for PE and other subjects.
- Regarding salaries, I presented in the last section my case for the enlarged role and responsibility for the rebranded PE teacher. They are trained but must be paid commensurate with their duties.
- The next three questions refer to the standards we delineated earlier. As noted, all states now have some quantified PE standards though no state, including Illinois, enforces their own standards. I did not want to put the ADs on the defense, though none left this question unanswered. I remain astounded that despite state standards being in place, they are treated as little more than "suggestions" and are dismissed if inconvenient.
- The next questions get at the heart of the matter: They attempt to verify that we are in fact spending money on a few to the detriment of many. As a nation, we seem to be of two minds regarding organized sports. We believe (again with no proof) that school sports serve a unique social benefit for the students, yet we seem happy to have only a portion of the students receiving this benefit. Not only was I keen to see what percentage of students were participating at all, I was also interested in how many are playing three sports, as the data shows this is directly proportional to health.
- With question 10, I was curious how many of the coaches were professional educators. We discussed earlier that children

often lose interest in organized sports due to poor coaching. It might be inferred that someone who has a degree in teaching would be more aware of the needs of student-athletes. I am also interested in what training these outside coaches received to qualify them for this job, though I did not feel I could bother the ADs for such complicated information on this survey.

- Finally, for the last two questions, I want to know how much money would be available if we were to offer PE and possibly some intramural sports for all students. My promise all along for my ideas regarding a rebranded PE was that it would be cost neutral. This data will give us the answers to whether the money is available for my PE assistants and the PE czar.

A word of appreciation: These ADs cared enough to take the time and they were brilliant. When they did not have an answer, they made that clear. As noted, they were candid when not following the state standards. Therefore, I believe this survey gives reliable data and a stark picture of the present situation in our nation's schools.

SURVEY SAYS . . .

Location: The great news here is we had responses from states across the country, including Hawaii though, alas, none from Alaska.

The School Sizes were also an excellent spread ranging from 31 to 3,200 students, with an average of just under 900.

The Number of Teachers on Staff averaged 1 for every 283 students. There was a range of 1:45 to a low of 1:840. We did not try to ascertain what other duties the teacher with only 45 students might have, just as we do not know what type of antianxiety counseling the teacher with 840 students is receiving! There were a number of schools that reported no dedicated PE teacher, the biggest of those with 800 students. There was also no clear correlation between pay and the number of students each teacher was responsible for.

The Average Salary was just north of $48,000, ranging from $25,000 for a school in Nebraska, to $125,000 for a New York City high school (though you might want to check the price of coffee and NYC housing before sending in your application).

PE Requirements: This is the question that I believe gets to the heart of physical identity. We need students to be active every day, though of course we know this does not happen. Earlier, we discussed state standards regarding one quantifiable aspect: time in PE class per week. We know the national standards as discussed in *Educating the Student Body: Taking Physical Activity and Physical Education to School* would be considered a minimum of 45 minutes a day for middle and high schoolers (Institute of Medicine, 2013). This equals 225 minutes a week, which some of our schools achieved. Such was not the case unfortunately, for the majority of our surveyed schools. The average PE time was 177 minutes per week. Not bad, you might think, as we have tried to keep the bar low throughout the book. But here is the problem: *No school that responded to our survey required PE for ALL students, EVERY day, for FOUR years.*

State Standards: This is data for which I am most impressed and appreciative, as it points to the honesty of our respondents. *A full 29% of ADs admitted to not following the state standards!* Now, if I was able to convince you of the value of these state standards as they impact our students' academic and physical health, and that there is little difference of opinion on this subject from state to state, you might well be appalled. But remember, the state standards, unlike the standards from the national study in *Educating the Student Body,* are literally all over the map. None are requiring the amount of activity we know children need for academic and health achievement. Also remember, this is the system we have chosen: local control of our school districts, no matter that many decide to ignore current science and knowledge. It is for this and other reasons that I will call for a PE czar to be in place in each state—so there can be some level of enforcement of the accepted standards of PE for every child, every day.

The Percentage That Play at Least One Varsity Sport: 50%. This is not a bad number (again, I have set the bar low), though I suspect it might be inflated as we had motivated ADs and missing in the survey was a big sampling of large, inner-city schools. Had more of these schools returned the survey, I suspect this number would get smaller, but perhaps I am being pessimistic.

The Percentage That Play Three Sports: 16%. If you are going to use organized sports for your fitness, it matters how many sports you play. There is a direct relationship to sports played and fitness. So are we okay with 16% of children being fit? I do not think so.

Percentage of Coaches Who Are Not Teachers on Staff: 47%. This may or may not be a good thing. The positive of bringing in coaches from outside the school is that students are exposed to different adults presumably with an interest in helping their education. Negatives might be the difficulty of gauging the level of expertise these coaches bring and, of course, the cost. What type of experience or credentials do these outside coaches have in dealing with teenagers? As noted, I did not ask the ADs to answer this question as the assessment of coaches can be extremely complicated and often contentious. Should they have many years of coaching that sport or have taken part in a credentialing process? Most of the time it has to do with relationships, which might be fine, though such relationships might exclude minorities, women, and others perhaps not in the "loop."

Percentage Spent on PE of the Total PE/Athletic Budget: 14%. Although one school reported spending the same amount on PE as they did on sports, *the vast majority spent far less on PE.* On average only 14% of the total sports and PE budget was spent on PE. There is a lot of money out there; it's just not being used for PE.

Other organizations have done research comparing PE spending with sports spending, finding similar results. A study done by *Shape america.org* broke down the physical education budget per student. The median physical education budget *per school year* in the United States was calculated to be $1,370 for high schoolers, $900 for those in middle school, and $460 for elementary school students, coming to an average of $764 per school year. This is not the annual budget toward equipment for each student—this is the cost per student when the teachers' salary, the physical plant, and other expenses were considered. Compare that to the $14,000 spending on high school students and $10,000 for middle schoolers toward athletics noted in the city cited above! Further data from this same study showed 60% of physical education teachers reported an *annual equipment budget* of under

$1,000 with 15% reporting an annual budget of $2,000 or more—that's the yearly PE budget for the *entire school*.

"When somebody says it's not about the money, it's about the money."

—H. L. Mencken

Although I did not find the breakdown that I sought in my examination of most school budget websites, I did come across some fascinating contributions. One of my favorites was a letter from a Maine high school AD. In it he recommends decreased funding of "freshman competition" in favor of "expanded athletics-based physical activity participation on the intramural level." When I saw this, I was super excited—here was a kindred spirit looking to broaden participation. Intramural sports are generally a far more efficient use of athletic department money compared to travel sports. My excitement did not last long, however, as he moved on to discuss establishing varsity boys and girls lacrosse, which had previously been a community sport (via Parks and Recreation). With all due respect, this is exactly the wrong direction to be taking with community club sports! Club teams are in fact the way things were and the way things should be going. For communities that support competitive high school sports programs, teams should play all comers. There should be agreements to allow competition against local club teams, no matter if some of these teams have players older than high school age, as long as the basics of safety, equipment, size, insurance, and other standards are met. We want to encourage *everyone* to be outside and active, not just students. Why should a club team not play a school team? Because this would confuse the state championship race? Please. In our present health crisis we simply cannot afford to have anything come between citizens and potentially fun activities.

As noted earlier, another of my concerns with organized school sports is that the cost to poorer schools is a proportionally greater part of their budget. A common estimate of the socioeconomic status of a school is the number of students receiving "free or reduced lunch." Although not perfect, this number varies depending on the household income and number of people in that household. According to the Federal Poverty Guidelines, a household income of below $45,000 for four people would allow a child to receive a reduced-price lunch, and below $31,000, a free lunch (Elementary and Secondary Education Act of 1965). Thus, when we ask two schools to field a baseball team, they both will have similar expenses regarding equipment, field maintenance, officiating, and so on, but the effect on the poorer school's budget would be greater. For example, Amundsen High School in Chicago, Illinois, which offers 25 sports to 1,200 students, has 83% of their students receiving free or reduced lunch (Amundsen High School). I would argue they would be at a disadvantage compared to Acalanes High School in Lafayette, California, a similar-sized school that also offers 25 sports to 1,300 students, but only 5% of their students receive free or reduced lunch (Explore Acalanes High School in Lafayette, CA). Clearly, Acalanes would be in a much stronger position to provide PE for all students, every day, and also be able to afford the 25 sports teams. The same I suspect cannot be said regarding Amundsen. Yet, as noted by the *Elementary and Secondary Education Act* discussed below, I would be hard pressed to understand how such an inequity jibes with "the opportunity to obtain a high-quality education" in both schools, especially as it pertains to physical education and perhaps other activities including art, drama, and music.

After you explore the school budgets in your own district, take a deep breath, and then try tackling some of the directives from our federal government. It will not take long to once again be "waist deep in the big muddy." Try, for example, the aforementioned Elementary and Secondary Education Act of 1965, as amended by the Every Student Succeeds Act (ESSA)–Accountability and State Plans (A Rule by the Education Department on 11/29/2016) (Elementary and Secondary Education Act of 1965). This is one of thousands of pieces of legislation regarding education that have been passed over the centuries, in this case noting:

The purpose of This Regulatory Action: On December 10, 2015, President Barack Obama signed the ESSA into law. The ESSA reauthorizes the ESEA, which provides federal funds to improve elementary and secondary education in the nation's public schools. The ESSA builds on ESEA's legacy as a civil rights law and *"seeks to ensure that every child, regardless of race, income, background, or where they live has the opportunity to obtain a high-quality education"* (italics mine).

Let that sink in for a moment. Does it strike anyone else as odd that in 2015 Americans needed to be spending energy on such legislation? It does, however, drive home my point. We are NOT, even today, giving children in America everything they deserve in a caring, egalitarian, and efficient fashion when it comes to education. We can do better, and we can do better with incredibly small effort. We can do better with no new money, no new technology, no new infrastructure, no new pedagogical knowledge. Progress can come simply with renewed allocation, will, determination, and most of all, the energy of the entire community. The numbers are clear. There is money. We simply need a redistribution so our schools fulfill the mission they were designed for. As discussed above, we need to harness the interest and caring of everyone in the school district—one does not have to be a teacher or parent to have a stake in the future of our children. Remember, our public schools are for teaching students, not for creating athletes to play in college or the Olympics. Our schools are not for running an entertainment division for the townspeople—they are there to educate the future townspeople.

MISSION STATEMENT

All schools have a mission statement. How about this:

> It is our mission at _____ School to provide a safe environment to nurture both the physical and cognitive aspects of our children's lives. When students leave here, they will be happy, fit, and intellectually curious. They will have the education and the desire to be caring citizens of the world, ready to work for the greater good.

We must stop giving any one aspect of student life, in this case school sports, more emphasis than it deserves. We must find the resolve to admit the present athletic system is not working for the vast majority of students. I make that statement knowing that taxpayers are resistant to making the money pie bigger. If this is the case, and knowing the importance of PE, we need to start taking money from the sports budget. And this makes sense, right? Money being distributed evenly, allocated for the greater good—in this case that good is the health of the next generation. Obviously, I am making an argument to the "haves": the vast majority of schools that have school sports. Those children in districts without PE *or* sports are in a much worse situation. This would not only need the efforts of the PE czar, but local politicians and community activists as such a condition is completely unacceptable in 21st-century America.

Though such decisions to reallocate money for the greater good may seem to go against years of development and myths regarding our organized sports system, they are not contrary to human evolution, and they are certainly not contrary to the original concept of school physical education. We must make a cultural shift away from a system that is far different than its original design and intention 100 years ago. We need a new system for the common good to balance the incredible changes of the last half century. This is necessary because while much has changed over the last 50 years, human beings have not. We still harbor the combination of primitive and cognitive aspects in our brains that require a combination of physical and intellectual work for a healthy existence. We need to stop asking students to be our court jesters, playing for our entertainment under the guise of education. We need a system that maintains physical identity in all students that does not depend on athletic skills and competition. We have the money. Now we must start a revolution that respects all students and fulfills our school's mission.

CHAPTER 5

Revolutionizing and Rebranding PE for Physical Identity

OUR SCHOOL IS IN MOTION: A SOCIAL CONTAGION

In this final chapter are plans for how we can achieve the goal of daily physical education (PE) classes in our public schools for the preservation and nurturing of physical identity. We have discussed the overwhelming evidence showing the benefits of daily exercise, yet it has not become the national norm. This is because no one has called for doing the hard work of demanding change. Let go of the mindset that "In a perfect world. . . ." We have a saying in the operating room that "perfect is the enemy of good." This is a labor of love, and we need to take the long view. Our first goal is to insist on "better" and with time achieve "good."

I want to introduce two mantras in this chapter: one for the adults and the other for the students. Here is the mantra for you new revolutionaries:

I have more power than I think!

Before you get scared and say that improving PE is a burden you might not want to carry, remember that this is only a positive for our students and children, with tons of data to support your efforts. Then there is this: We are truly talking about the physical and mental health of the next generation. In this chapter we are going to first establish some specific goals for our rebranded PE program using evidence-based research as our guide. We will then provide a template for a month of PE classes for elementary, middle, and high schoolers that get our heart rates up and create the "brain fertilizer" discussed by Dr. Ratey (Ratey, 2013). Finally, we will discuss specifically how the PE revolution can come to your school district.

GOALS FOR THE REBRANDED PE

My belief for what today's PE should look like, and my belief for participation in most school activities, can be summarized in the students' mantra:

Our school is in motion!

This is the attitude we want our students to aspire to both at school and at home, no matter what the assignment. Students should give their best effort and show high energy in every subject because they know the teachers and entire school staff have their best interests at heart. No two-class system of good students and bad students, or athletes and nonathletes. Children *want* to be in motion. This means we do not have to break habits ("Get off the computer.") because they never stopped doing what their primitive brain asked for (play!). Their behaviors are automatic. We do not need to convince them that getting outside, running, swimming, cycling, and being part of the natural world is good for them—they know this. We simply need to make it easier for them. This not only includes PE every day but an environment, a neighborhood, a town, that allows easy access to play: bike paths, open gyms, playgrounds, walking trails, swimming pools—creating real competition for the video screen. We must give up often unsubstantiated fears that the only way to protect our children is to lock them inside. By letting them be children, by letting them simply play, they also glean all the social benefits we discussed in Chapter 1, including starting friendships, problem solving, flexibility, and cooperation. Then, if we can somehow make getting on that screen inconvenient (and yes administrators and parents—I'm looking at you!), we have a strong foundation for our revolution. We know the game manufacturers and ultra-processed food makers are worthy enemies. We must tilt the scales in favor of our physical identity with every means available.

Although making an attitude a "goal" perhaps bends some of the rules of goal setting we emphasize in sport psychology, such reimagining is exactly where we need to start the PE revolution. We create definable goals for athletes. Since I do not consider any of my hunter-gatherer brethren nonathletes, we need to have definable physical goals for everyone. The most common acronym athletes use when discussing goal setting is "SMART" (O'Neill, 2008):

SMART Goal Setting

- Specific
- Measurable
- Attainable
- Realistic
- Time-sensitive

The attitude goal of *"our school is in motion"* can be made specific, measurable, attainable, and is imminently realistic. As we all know, there is a time factor of exactly 13 years to achieve this goal. If we harken back to our discussion of the primitive brain, we know that being busy, curious, and in motion is *what children do*. We are simply guides for their primitive animal circuitry. Let's see what this might look like in action.

"S" = Specific

Elementary School. For elementary students, proper PE looks like having the playground and, in bad weather, the gym, open and supervised when the students arrive at school. For those without dedicated gymnasiums, a couple of classrooms or a cafeteria with the furniture pushed aside can work as well. A few balls, jump ropes, or painted lines and presto!—the children will use their imagination for the rest. Arriving to school early should be encouraged, and perhaps even an expectation facilitated by arrangements with bus companies, to get the juices flowing. This is simply the equivalent of an adult going for an early morning run or fitness class. Ideally, there would be a faculty member there able to encourage some "functional movement patterns," but ultimately nothing should stand in the way of motion. Importantly, players should not be worried about losing a ball or scuffing the floor, as these are great problems to have. How wonderful would it be to hear the complaints at a school board meeting: "We use our play equipment so much the students are wearing it out!" "We have to repaint the hop-scotch and Four-Square lines outside every year!" "Our custodial crew needs to resurface the gym floor to deal with all the traffic." "The students come to homeroom already sweating." This early morning play time is exactly what we established at one of our local schools on a more formal basis, and the response from parents, teachers, and children was overwhelmingly positive.

Play before class will have the students ready for the first bout of lessons. Ideally midmorning the same day, a formal PE period will follow. This is the time to help the youngsters develop a happy emotional connection to "organized" activity. What we need to avoid in this controlled chaos is winners and losers. For the younger children this is even more vital. They will need less coaxing than the older students to get moving and have fun. At this level, we establish the child's self-worth and what we call in the sport psychology field "self-efficacy."

Self-efficacy is a phrase developed by Albert Bandura that refers to a person's sense of being able to do something they think they can do (Bandura, 1977). In other words, if a child believes they can accomplish a task—or even has a chance to accomplish that task—they will be more inclined to try. In the case of PE, if children are encouraged and given challenges that are within their ability—or perhaps just beyond their ability—they will attempt them. An activity can be challenging but still appropriate for the level the children are at, with the emphasis on letting the children *play*. Activities encourage motion and fun, with the teachers and fellow students making sure everyone is involved—no one sits on the sidelines. What the PE teacher does not need to do at this age is a lot of skill teaching. For example, hitting a baseball or softball is a daunting task in the best of times (just ask any major league hitter!). Trying to teach almost any sports skills in this short period of time is not going to help many students, as they will not succeed and potentially get frustrated. On the other hand, almost everyone can participate in kicking a ball, hanging from bars, and balancing something on their head while running around obstacles. This is the age and time where PE is being branded. It needs to be a brand of simplicity, trust, and fun. This is how we will maintain physical identity and interest in PE for the long haul. Except for words of caring and encouragement, they need play, not lectures. As you will see later in our suggestions for classes, we are not opposed to throwing, hitting, and catching balls—the emphasis though should never waver from motion and smiles!

Ideally, students will make the concept of *our school is in motion* as part of their personal philosophy. Internalizing this concept can color their daily activities. They do not look for the easiest or shortest route somewhere. They do not wait for the next person to chase down a ball that went over the fence or pick up the stray paper. They do it themselves because *our school is in motion*. They make the effort. They sweat. They laugh. They encourage each other. When health and toughness are part of their physical identity, this attitude develops and feeds on itself.

Middle School. For middle school students, activities can reflect their maturation and thus a more academic connection to physical fitness. These youths (ages 11–14) are at an important transition that can tax the imagination of the PE professional. This might be the toughest group for teachers, just as it is a tough group for me in sports medicine and sport psychology, and tough for parents! A 14-year-old might have the physical maturity of an 11- or 17-year-old depending on where they are regarding puberty. As most adolescents' bodies are starting to mature, this is a good age to start teaching training techniques for general fitness.

In *Knee Surgery: The Essential Guide to Total Knee Recovery* (O'Neill, 2008), I discuss the "muscle qualities" of balance, coordination, flexibility, strength, endurance, speed, and quickness. You will see examples of these qualities in the sample classes below. Middle school is a great time to introduce these concepts, as students are developing the tools and knowledge for a lifetime of fitness. We can now put names on what the elementary students were doing simply as play—squats, planks, pull-ups (with bands!), push-ups, stretches, and so on— movements that are the building blocks for all activities. The children will have been influenced by what they see in the media—take that lead. Let them make up their own contests and games using these movements. Anything they are excited about that fits in the basic plan can be offered, allowing something for everyone. Having the children participate in class planning is often referred to as "student voice and choice" (Larmer, 2016). In classes where students have no voice or choice, they can feel powerless with always being told what to study and what to do. This can often lead to disinterest and the worst result: no learning and no fun. In PE, they can be empowered to make their own rules so long as they are moving. My friend tells me the reason he loves coaching this age group is that the students make him laugh every day. Although challenging, middle school classes should be the most entertaining for the PE teachers and assistants.

At the risk of breaking my preference for low-tech solutions, a good use of a smartphone would be to help the students with their techniques using visual feedback (and children this age love seeing themselves on screen!). Children are much better at "modeling" behavior than adults. They can see something and replicate it easily with their supple joints and lack of bad habits. Giving video feedback on a squat or kick will go a long way toward improvement and interest. Again, I want to emphasize that while technology can be used as a supplement and tool, it is hardly necessary. What is necessary is the enthusiasm, caring, and energy of the *entire* school staff. No fancy equipment is going to maintain a child's physical identity. Physical identity comes from the primitive brain, and that primitive brain wants to *move*. Motion does not cost money—just ask Isaac Newton.

One thing about feedback—it should always be positive and geared toward progress. The John Wooden method of feedback—telling his players "this is what you're doing, this is how I want you to do it, this is how you get there"—is time tested and not demeaning (Wooden & Jamison, 2018). PE teachers need to channel their inner "surfer dude" when it comes to feedback. Feedback should be positive and high energy, but still constructive and never vapid. A child knows when they are not giving full effort. If a teacher has low expectations, the students will lower themselves to that expectation, and the result will be an ineffective program. Rebranded PE emphasizes simplicity, trust, and fun. Students are there to learn, and the vast majority will value adult attention and opinion. A PE teacher must never lose belief in their students' potential.

Middle school is also a great age for cycling, as the children are more skilled and keen to be independent. PE expert Niall Moyna thinks every child should learn to walk (check!), swim, and ride a bike, and I could not agree more. In inner-city schools, the PE czar could make a deal with the city bike program to use their machines (and in shop class students could help repair them, as we always want to be looking for "value-added products"). The students would get to learn to ride a bike and start an activity that will be with them the rest of their lives. They would also learn about the local community, traffic patterns, and safety. The number of cycling games are endless.

The benefits of daily PE also do not stop when the students leave school. There is good research showing that children are *more active* after school on PE days, not less active. (They do not go home "tired." Have people who say that ever had a dog?) Rather than ask what students did on their summer vacations, homeroom teachers should be asking the class what they did for activity after school *yesterday*.

A PE teacher responds:

> As a middle school gym teacher, I am getting kids that cannot move with any efficiency. Similar to a seventh-grade child who cannot read, my students cannot move, and the first half of the year is spent teaching movements significantly more basic than a squat or plank.

High School. When I was a senior in high school, some friends and I were heading out to spend the night on the beach. This was frowned upon (okay, it was illegal), so stealth was key. At one point, a wrestling match broke out and the grapplers were told to "stop acting like idiots." Another friend noted, "We're 17 years old, we're supposed to be idiots." There is a lot going on in high school, and while we expect a level of maturity and decorum, these young people are still adolescents (and sometimes idiots!). On the other hand, they also want to be treated as adults, which we can oblige on many levels. Adolescents are more and more focused on sexuality, and this energy can be used. There are multiple models for exercise circuits with dumbbells, air squats, burpees, jump ropes, and so on, that people pay big money for. This is time and cash well spent because in 30–45 minutes a day (the length of a gym class), adults get a workout that can actually change their physiques. Not only do they feel more attractive, they are fitter for everyday activities, just as the students will feel better and fitter heading back to class. Now before getting your eyes stuck, remember that we have ideally developed trust with the students in the previous 9 years (assuming they had daily PE with certified PE teachers)! They have seen the benefits of PE since elementary school. I appreciate if we were to start this program today at the high school level it would sadly be met with resistance. This is why we must start in the elementary grades and never let their physical identity lapse. Ever.

An inner-city high school PE teacher responds:

> While on the whole students choose to attend my high school
> as it is a magnet school, there are still huge socioeconomic,
> cultural, and behavioral differences that can lead to multiple
> issues. Motivating the students is like "pulling teeth." The
> students' number one priority is the phone, and I believe they
> are essentially addicted. The school has to a large extent given up
> on enforcing the "no phone" policy, and students are Facetiming
> friends in the same building during the school day. With the
> advent of ear buds, I have now taken to asking them to remove
> any hats so I know they are not on the phone!
>
> And yes—basic skills are lacking in every activity we attempt.
> I had kids show up for softball tryouts not knowing they needed a
> glove. *I mean, really?*

One of the schools I worked with, Burke Mountain Academy, is for those students interested in ski racing (About Us, n.d.). Multiple graduates go on to compete for the U.S. Ski Team, and a point of pride is that when they arrive on the national team, "Burkies" know how to *train*. They leave Burke knowing proper strength-training techniques, such as how to do the most basic of all exercises: the squat. This should be the goal of every high school PE program: that the graduates leave understanding movement fundamentals they will use the rest of their lives. Not only will this allow them to enter any health club around the world knowing how to get a good workout, but just as importantly, it will allow them to pull the engine out of a tractor or carry that couch up the stairs without hurting their back!

Most PE classes in senior high should engage a combination of muscle qualities with a mix of aerobic ("cardio"), strength, flexibility, coordination, and so on. This not only helps train these different qualities, but it keeps all players involved. Although ideally we "train our weaknesses"—that is, if you are tight you should be doing more flexibility, not less—people do not want to do only things they struggle with, especially teenagers. A varied circuit setup allows everyone to feel competent at times, while still being challenged at other times (self-efficacy). What we do not need to be doing at this stage is worrying about skills like serving a tennis ball. Every person will hopefully be doing squats for fitness at some point in their life. They need to know how to squat. Tennis is great, as long as they are whacking and moving, not worrying about how to keep score.

We all have an image of the worst "athlete" in the school. Too big, too small, skinny or fat, pants that did not stay up no matter what, bad shoes, and so on. How do we keep that child's physical identity? How do we tilt the playing field in their direction so they see success and pleasure in gym class? In addition to the concepts of simplicity, trust, and fun emphasized earlier, one of the ways is to not design gym class as a series of skilled games. These do not increase fitness for the students, but only widen the athlete vs. nonathlete divide. Ideally, get the czar involved. If soccer or basketball is played, it should be made fun, not a competition to the death. Three on three, a decent distance between goals so the folks are running, no goalie, bringing the hoop low for "dunking," requiring everyone to touch the ball each time down the field, everything fast fast fast, are just some examples of what the games should look like (see below for much more).

Even more so at this age we want to let the students suggest their own games, as long as bodies are in motion, breathing hard, and showing effort. We touched on student leaders previously. With the dearth of PE teachers, this is a great place to involve older students in organizing themselves. A student could be teaching a dance or yoga class in one room, while others head out for a run. But it cannot only be the "jocks" doing the organizing. There needs to be a rotation so everyone is put in such a position, as well as a culture of respect so that all will be listened to (voice and choice). This again leads back to our discussion of self-efficacy. High schoolers might be incentivized by allowing student-led classes as an extension of the PE assistant, to fulfill part of their PE requirement. Every student will be in some type of position requiring organization as adults, even if just as parents. Shouldn't we be teaching them this now, in a nurturing and positive environment? Such a supervisory role will further internalize their physical identities and take some of the pressure off the busy PE teacher, or in many schools, the classroom teacher asked to teach PE.

A high school coach replies:

> The athlete/nonathlete divide is a significant impediment to keeping kids off the field and seems to have worsened as my career progressed. Many students simply do not respond to the structured sports environment their parents often put them in. That's why I think yoga, dance, and other alternative activities are vital. Or if they must do a sport, such as in some private schools, get them involved with track and cross-country running—sports that do not necessitate brilliant skills but have the motion and team comradery. Athletes seem to understand the value of their bodies, and at this age, body image, especially in girls, can be a huge issue. For these and other reasons, we somehow must ensure that all students maintain that joy of connection with their physical being. When they are old like me, their activities should be limited by available time, not by heart disease or knee arthritis.

Importantly, *nothing suggested in our program involves expensive equipment or technology*. This thinking is not new. Such ideas have existed in the past and are happening now in enlightened schools. There is no reason your school cannot be one of them. In a proper PE class, everyone is in motion because this is what our school does, this is what humans do—not just athletes, but all human animals. So much can be accomplished and so many calories can be burned in 30 or 40 minutes that the students will be keen for biology class, not squirming in their seats (Zientarski, 2015). Good PE is not only a great "pump primer" for academics, but after going hard for half an hour, come lunchtime youngsters actually *want* to put some healthy nutrition in their bodies, not junk food.

When discussing roadblocks to PE, one of the topics that came up in multiple forms was the attitude of the staff: PE teachers' attitudes toward their students, non–PE teachers' attitudes toward PE teachers, administration's attitudes toward standardized testing, cafeteria workers' attitudes to healthy food, and so on. Rebranded PE starts with the teacher and the principal and must be passed up and down. Getting the entire staff on board will be welcomed by the vast majority simply because happier students make everybody happy—another social contagion. Of course, there might always be an Eeyore. Too bad for them, but hopefully with time, they will be positively contaminated also.

"M" = Measurable

Make *"our school is in motion"* the mantra and primary goal, and youthful energy will carry the day. Key to the program I am proposing is that we are not talking about "traditional" physical education as most of us know it. This is where the "measurable" aspects of *our school is in motion* come in. How did people like Tony Horton (P90X) and John Foley (Peloton) get rich and famous? They found a way to make burning calories and getting fit *fun*. They developed quantifiable programs that appeal to our primitive brain. They promised that if people committed themselves they would see measurable results. In the case of Peloton, your own work output numbers are clearly displayed in front of you. For more motivation, there is a "leaderboard" that shows how you stack up against the others taking the class. These two people, smart though they are, did not discover anything new. They simply put together a scheme that every day fires up our primitive brain. PE teachers learn in their university classes what appeals to the primitive brains of students K–12. These teachers deserve the freedom to use that knowledge. Surely students should not be having nightmares about shaving 5 seconds off their time for the 400-meter run the next morning, but they do benefit from seeking measurable results. Rebranded PE is egalitarian in that everyone participates on an equal level, though clearly each child's output and results will differ. *The main measure is effort.* Although this effort can be quantified with technology, self-reports, taking a pulse, and teacher observations can be just as relevant. Just as when a student is put in a supervisory role, even the more physically challenged students will most often rise to the occasion, not drag people down. I witnessed this every time I took to the slopes with my middle school ski group. The classmates encouraged each other, though not everyone was a fast skier. This is what leadership is about, and facilitating this is part of the PE teacher's role. For teachers who need help, this is the perfect opportunity for a good principal or the czar to step up.

"A" = Attainable

One of the research papers I wrote had to do with the "social contagion" effect, a phrase I used earlier (O'Neill, 2008). We have all seen social contagion on some level, with the Salem Witch Trials being an extreme example that most schoolchildren have read about. I attended a wedding years ago at the Salem Witch Museum, as the museum would rent space at night to help fund the exhibits. I learned that night that some 20 people were put to death until clearer minds prevailed (yes—I should have been dancing—it was our last date!). Courteous driving and not littering are social contagions on a more local level. I became interested in this concept as it was my concern that an injury to one athlete could "contaminate" other athletes, causing them to change their tactics, possibly resulting in a higher rate of injury ("injury contagion"). For example, if one ski racer crashes at a tight turn, do the other racers who change their line to avoid falling, possibly put themselves at greater risk? Making activity and fitness an attainable, positive, "social contagion" works if one can develop the school culture to foster it. Let us look at three examples of schools that created a culture of fitness and their potential attainability for other schools.

La Sierra High School, Carmichael, California. La Sierra High School has taken on an almost mythical status in the world of PE and was a model for some of President Kennedy's Council on Physical Fitness ideas (John F. Kennedy Library and Museum, n.d.). In the late 1950s, the football coach Stan LeProtti (who was also the athletic director—arguably a good or bad thing) developed a program of PE for the *boys* (though the school was coed) that involved at least 15 minutes of *competitive* exercise a day. There are films of these classes that can be found on YouTube and need to be seen to be believed. You will not see that many six packs at a beer distributor! Boys were segregated in various fitness groups depicted by different colored shorts. Judging from the films, they rarely wore shirts.

The exercises performed in the La Sierra videos would fit in fine with PE classes from 100 years ago and are great for developing basic fitness and burning calories. As opposed to today's emphasis on moderate to vigorous physical activity (MVPA), the focus at La Sierra was on strength and functional motion. Negative aspects of the program are strong elements of social engineering and machismo, as this was taking place in the early days of rock and roll, the pill, and the "hippie" revolution. A *Look Magazine* article from January 1962 notes, "The program, in sum, not only builds physical fitness, but good Americans" (Theisen, n.d.). Female students did not become involved until years later. Despite its weaknesses, the program went national with some 4,000 high schools eventually participating, though it is not clear how long either La Sierra or the other schools continued such an aggressive program. La Sierra closed in 1983 (Welcome La Sierra H.S. Longhorns!, n.d.).

There are certainly many things I like about the La Sierra program—the emphasis on hard but simple exercises, being part of a motivating group, measuring the students' progress, the fact that they did not need fancy, expensive equipment, and the concept of daily effort. These qualities are something we see with programs like P90X. Such programs emphasize hard work and consistency to create healthy changes. If you do not raise your heart rate, stress your muscles, and do it 5 or 6 days a week, you will not see the fitness gains most people (and their doctors) seek.

What I do not think would work with the La Sierra program today is the crazy high intensity and the strict stratification denoted by the different colored shorts. High repetitions, intensity, and competition eventually wear people out, making such a program generally unsustainable. I am in favor of meeting in the middle to set up a high-energy program with clear measurable gains that might be more individual, not as public, and hopefully more fun! Obviously, the social elements of La Sierra's grooming, "manliness," and exclusion of women do not belong in a modern PE class.

One of the things I did not see in the old films from La Sierra High School are the boys who did not have a six-pack. Where are these folks? Are they somewhere getting a good workout? Yes, they had the benefit of not being fed toxic, ultra-processed foods, but there must have been some laggards. Are they too maximizing their time? A proper rebranded PE program raises all boats.

Holderness School, Holderness, New Hampshire. The Holderness School is in my hometown, and one I have been associated with as a team doctor for many years. As luck would have it, I also served on an advisory panel at Holderness as they sought to revamp their athletic programs and facilities in the midst of writing this book. The timing could not have been better, as there were two-dozen minds in one room discussing many of the issues presented in these pages. Although Holderness is still referred to in many parts of town as the "Boys' School," it is actually a private college preparatory high school that has been around since 1879 and coed since the late 1970s (Holderness, n.d.). Though a private school is not a perfect metaphor, Holderness epitomizes the values we would hope to see in every school: *a commitment to both the physical and academic achievement for all students.* Holderness has a "three-sport model," where students are involved with (mostly) outdoor activities throughout the school year. This model is more and more uncommon, even in private schools, just as daily PE is uncommon in public schools. Holderness does not offer PE per se but requires sports participation instead. The sports are 6 days a week and only as competitive as each student wants them to be. In other words, if someone wants to play basketball but has never strapped on a pair of high-topped sneakers, they might have a fun 4-year career on the junior varsity. Noncompetitive sports such as recreational skiing, rock climbing, and other activities are offered in this school on the edge of the White Mountains. Almost all sports have an aerobic component, and classes resume after the daily break for athletics. Participation, teamwork, and sportsmanship are truly emphasized.

The part of a Holderness athletic experience that is incredibly impressive, and easily replicable in any school, is the attitude of the staff. Although most schools cannot replicate the playing fields and rural surroundings of Holderness, attitude is something that can not only be established in every school but is contagious. Teachers often double as coaches, but even more importantly, every administrator, groundskeeper, admissions officer, and so on knows that physical activity is a part of the school day, that it is part of the school *culture*. The balance of physical and mental work maintains the entire student body's strong physical identity.

Naperville Central High School, Naperville, Illinois. Perhaps the poster child for PE in a public school today is Naperville Central High School in Illinois. The brilliant thing about the program at Naperville, and something we should always look for to guide our recommendations, is that it is *scientifically based*. Naperville is the school that also served as a talisman for the push in Illinois to recommend daily "enhanced" PE for every student in the state. Although Illinois admits on its website that they have not yet achieved the statewide K–12 participation asked for, they have a good carrot in Naperville.

As with the program at La Sierra, it is worth a quick YouTube search to see what the PE classes look like in Naperville (Need to Know, 2011). The students are in the constant motion I have been calling for. Many are on a program of doing moderate to vigorous physical activity (MVPA) before school or, ideally, before their toughest classes. One thing that stands out is their use of technology. The "gym" is filled with spin bikes, treadmills, and other high-tech (read: expensive) equipment. It looks far more like an exclusive exercise club in a major city than a suburban high school. They put the technology to good use and actually measure the student's pulse to ensure they are spending the right amount of time in the predetermined exercise "zone." After the "prescribed" bout of exercise, the child is deemed ready for a day of academics. Naperville has been able to quantify significant gains on standardized math and other tests. And this makes sense. Despite the numerous websites, puzzles, games, and other "tricks" directed mostly at older folks to keep their brains healthy, the strongest data for avoiding the ravages of Alzheimer's is not working the brain; it is working the body (Ahlskog et al., 2011). If the best way to hold off Alzheimer's is exercise, it should make complete sense that this connection of brain health and "below the neck" health would manifest throughout life.

What Naperville also created, though he was not referred to as such, was a PE czar in the form of teacher Paul Zientarski. Mr. Zientarski is exactly the high-energy, confident, and charismatic leader we need in our PE czars. He is very *intentional* regarding his program: His intention is to make better students. As Mr. Zientarski makes clear, after

PE periods, students do not come to class "hyped-up," but they come ready to learn (Zientarski, 2015). Additionally, and one of the real keys that we would hope to see with any good PE program, the obesity rate at this school is far below the state and national averages.

John Ratey, MD, a psychiatrist from Harvard Medical School, heard about the program in Naperville and has become a huge advocate. He describes their fitness-based PE program as creating "brain fertilizer," citing research showing actual changes in positive neurotransmitter production and cellular growth in the brain of the students doing aggressive PE. In his book *Spark: The Revolutionary New Science of Exercise and the Brain*, he gives a detailed scientific explanation for the benefits of programs such as that at Naperville (2013). For those of you interested in learning more about the physiology of exercise and its effect on brain functioning, this book is a must read.

One concern I have regarding the Naperville program is whether it is sustainable into adulthood. The school requires the youngsters to give hard physical efforts, sometimes before school. Naperville is not just concerned with the student's future health, but is concerned with academics *now*. My fear is that some students will associate exercise with high heart rate intervals and pain. If a student gets her heart rate up to 90% of its maximum for algebra class, what happens when algebra is over? All children must identify as active, primitive human animals, and keep active because it is a physical need, otherwise the results of any program will not be sustainable. Though we described the success of programs such as Peloton as necessitating hard work, there is a line between big efforts and agony. The fear that exercise will hurt is an excuse that many people use to *not* exercise at all. But there is also a line between health benefits and pain. Finding this zone and working within it allows one to look forward to exercise, not dread it.

My other issue with Naperville is the heavy dependence on technology. As someone who enjoys the science of fitness, this approach would work for me if it were available when I was in high school. I suspect most students there are already using technology as part of their lives and having it in the gym is a logical extension. The downside to this model is the expense of heart rate monitors, spin cycles, kinetic strength machines, aerobic assessments, and so on. Lower technology methods such as simply checking the pulse, learning breathing techniques, marking perceived exertion scales, and the use of "old school" exercises can achieve the same end and are thus available immediately at any school, with no financial outlay. *Allowing the students to think they need a machine to get healthy goes against my sensibility and theory that we need children to get outside to maintain their physical identity as human animals.* As the inner-city PE teacher reminded us earlier, technology can often work against us.

These complaints regarding the Naperville program are minor in the overall picture. I would hope, as seems to be the case, that these students associate exercise with success, energy, discipline, and fond memories of how their body responds to physical stress so they will continue being active throughout their lives.

"R" = Realistic

We are now up to the "R" in our SMART goal setting: realistic. One criticism of the Naperville program is that it takes place in a prosperous suburban school that has significant resources to put toward a program with pools, bikes, and other cool equipment. I completely appreciate, however, that it is not *realistic* to enact such an expensive program in most school districts. Naperville might be where we all want to be, but we need a plan that will save lives *now*, not wait for perfection. The medical equivalent of this would be a novel surgery for a common ailment, but due to special equipment it could only be performed in a few hospitals. We need programs that can be established not just in Naperville or in Holderness—we need programs that can be started nationwide immediately.

Although there might not exist the ideal physical space, this should never be a reason for not having the will to start some type of rebranded PE. This is where the PE czar comes in. One of the jobs of the state PE czar is to act as or train a "Paul Zientarski" in every school. These people exist—they just need to be given the credentials and freedom to work. We talked about the importance of also getting community leaders involved. In poorer schools, using the energy of programs like "Teach for America" (Teach for America, n.d.) and the leadership and largesse of a local professional sports team might be considered. But whether this help does or does not become available, it cannot excuse the lack of progress at any location. "Making do" is what has turned countless start-up companies into successes. A skier friend of mine says that the best snow in the world is what you are skiing on. In other words, you cannot spend your life paralyzed to act, wishing for "perfect." The best gym in the world might be that revamped classroom. Yes, treadmills and heart-rate monitors are nice, but jump ropes and perceived level of exertion scales with a finger on the wrist work just as well, without the expense and maintenance.

How wonderful would it be if a school an hour away in inner-city Chicago could match the results of Naperville without any bells and whistles? In fact, this can be the case, working off teacher, staff, and student energy. Another success story is from our neighbor to the north. In Saskatoon, Canada, at City Park Collegiate High School, they instituted an aggressive aerobic-based exercise program. And this is not a school for the rich and famous. City Park Collegiate is described as a "school of last resort" for children who "haven't been able to make it anywhere else" (Brain Gain, 2008). Fifty percent of the students have attention-deficit/hyperactivity disorder as well as other challenges. Despite these disadvantages, bringing in a daily exercise program to the school made a huge difference in academic achievement. These are the same issues we see in poor districts all over the world.

Please do not think I am a Pollyanna regarding this subject. I appreciate, among other roadblocks, that teacher shortages or teacher "maldistribution" are real issues (Busey, 2011). However, bringing in rebranded PE is not only *realistic* but is actually more necessary in these schools. For example, the vicious cycle of teacher attrition in the inner cities (40% over 5 years in one study), leading to poor academics leading to misbehavior leading to student attrition is real but will not be ended with old methods and old energy (ibid.). Whether we are talking about rich or poor, city or country, the precepts are the same for all schools because all students have the same physical needs.

One more note about creating a revolution. When we discussed roadblocks to a rebranded PE program earlier, one of the issues was the apathy of the students. This is because we have allowed their physical identity to lapse. Although today's 17-year-old might sadly be a lost cause, if we start in kindergarten with daily PE, once they reach high school, having been brought up in a rebranded PE culture, they will be "all-in" because *they are in motion*. At that point, exercise will be part of their physical identity, and importantly, part of a social contagion.

Nothing makes me sadder than hearing why we cannot accomplish something as simple as this in America, Ireland, Canada, or essentially any country that is in an obesity crisis. As stated, the money is there. I have no doubt that companies and organizations will line up to get involved, and using professional revenue ideas such as selling naming rights to the field or gym should not be dismissed. What schools cannot do is wait around for fancy equipment and facilities. This is a quality-of-life issue. This is a public health issue. There should be no delaying, as such measures will benefit the health of the next generation. With positive feedback from parents, teachers, and test scores once they see the benefits of PE, other community members will jump into action to be part of the success. We saw this with the introduction of something as simple as stand-up desks at one of our local elementary schools. After introducing the desks to one classroom, there was a story in the local paper exclaiming the enthusiasm of the students participating. Soon after, a donation was made to expand the program, and now almost every classroom offers stand-up desks. Viva la revolution!

"T" = Time Sensitive

Our physical education revolution to nurture physical identity needs to happen in the 13 or so years we have to influence our students. The brilliant work they are doing at City Park Collegiate and in other locations has proven to be effective yet does not seem to be catching fire worldwide. Something is stopping other school districts from doing the same thing. We are hoping with this book, educators will realize this model is possible in their school without tons of money, without technology, and without a beautiful physical plant. The rebranded PE revolution is possible when the staff of each school makes the decision *every day* that *our school is in motion.*

One of the Holy Grails to making this rebranded PE work is not allowing the building of walls between the so-called athlete and non-athlete. We need to allow the most uncoordinated "nerds" to keep in touch with their primitive brain. In Chapter 4 we saw how a minority of the student population is playing an organized sport and thus considers themselves athletes. It is the rest, the majority, that we must keep on board with fun PE.

PE class is like the operating room and time is of the essence. There is nothing that is neutral during surgery. Every move is either positive or negative. When a patient is under anesthesia, they are essentially being poisoned and we must limit that as much as possible. Children in PE class will either get their heart rate up, have fun, and stimulate their brains, or they will lose self-esteem and precious time to release positive neurotransmitters. We need a surgeon's sense of urgency and intention every minute, in every PE class, every day.

SAMPLE CURRICULA

This is where the "rubber sneaker soles meet the gym floor." PE teacher Elizabeth Savage has put together a program that can be re-created in any school, in any location, with minimal equipment. She provides a daily program for 4 weeks at each school level. These programs can serve as a template for your own students and hopefully will stimulate your own creativity for other exercises. Remember that the only rules for the daily exercises is that they must raise heart rates, they must be egalitarian, and they must be fun! We will not go into gory detail regarding the following exercises as the shorthand used should be familiar to most PE professionals. Take a look at all three levels as in addition to some crossover, there are some great ideas that can pertain to students of any age. We would also welcome any questions or comments, and our contact information can be found at the end of the book. We use the word "gym" or "field," but of course this could just as easily say classroom or parking lot. The space used should never be a constraint. Great thanks to Avery Feigenbaum and his "Animals in Motion" program for his input (Faigenbaum & Bruno, 2017).

Elementary Curriculum

ENGAGEMENT IN PHYSICAL ACTIVITY:

These movements are designed to get students excited about the task at hand. Participate in moderate to vigorous aerobic physical activity and muscle strength activities each day. There can be some lighter days to avoid burnout that might focus more on such qualities as flexibility and coordination. "Instant Activities" are designed to engage students as they enter the gym (or field).

HEALTH AND SKILL-RELATED FITNESS:

Classify activities as light, medium, difficult with the focus on heart rate (wrist pulse) and physiological response to activity (e.g., perceived exertion scale). Each day's activities are broken down into Warm-Up, Workout, and Activity.

BENEFITS OF ACTIVITY:

Activities with friends (and family!) should be challenging, new, fun, and allow for self-expression. They all make the heart, lungs, and muscles stronger so children are better prepared for more demanding games and exercises later in life.

SOCIAL INTERACTION:

Be safe, cooperate, and encourage peers. This is where the things we have attributed to sports—fair play, camaraderie, and effort—can all be taught in a safe, nurturing, and less competitive environment.

WEEK 1—DAY 1

ENGAGEMENT IN PHYSICAL ACTIVITY:

Instant Activity:

Have four cones in each corner of the gym. As students enter, give them a color cone to report to. Each cone will have a picture of a body weight exercise.

Examples:

1. Hold a push-up position on your knees or toes.
2. Jumping jacks or ski jumps.
3. Mountain climbers.
4. High knees.

HEALTH-RELATED FITNESS:

Warm-Up:

Whistle Walk: Walk around space, and when the whistle blows go a bit faster to open space.

Workout: Walk around the outside of the gym, and when the whistle blows once skip, and if it blows twice run. Three whistles will indicate walking again. Continue for 3–4 minutes.

Activity: Walk the inside of the gym. Two taggers will be running, and if they tag you, you can run and also help tag.

Activity Focus: Pace and moving in space

BENEFITS OF ACTIVITY:

Weekly Mini Lesson: Heart Rate
Benefits of getting heart rate up during activity

SOCIAL INTERACTION:

Keep eyes up and move safely in space.

WEEK 1—DAY 2

ENGAGEMENT IN PHYSICAL ACTIVITY:

Instant Activity:

Students enter the gym and go to cone groups from Day 1. Remind them of color or make new groups. At each cone they can run in place to increase heart rate. If they need to rest, they should be taught to control breathing with big deep slow breaths, especially on the exhale (slow count 4 in, slow count 5 out), and then continue to run in place.

HEALTH-RELATED FITNESS:

Warm-Up:

Popsicle Stick Relay. Put several pop sticks in the middle of the gym. Students will be in cone groups from Instant Activity. On the signal one from each cone group will run and pick up a pop stick. The next player goes to get one when his/her teammate returns. This continues until all sticks are picked up. Reverse game so that students put sticks back in the middle.

  Heart Rate Mini Lesson—pulse points—test at beginning of activity and end.

  Pulse is the impulse of the heart contraction and can be felt anywhere you can feel an artery, though the wrist is generally the easiest and safest.

Workout:

Running from cone to cone to increase heart rate. Slow on the short side and fast on the long side of the gym. How many laps can you do in 2 minutes?

Activity:

Race Track. Run the track until the whistle blows. When you hear the whistle, you can try to pass as many "cars" as possible. Try to count your passes.

Activity Focus: Heart Rate

SOCIAL INTERACTION:

Cheer for your team. Learn to high five at the end of games—both teammates and other teams.

WEEK 1—DAY 3

ENGAGEMENT IN PHYSICAL ACTIVITY:

Instant Activity:

Meet students at the door of the gym. Have them Bear Crawl to either side of gym (cone on side or cone standing). This will set up the Warm-Up.

HEALTH-RELATED FITNESS:

Warm-Up:

Cone Flip. Half the students go to the cone that is standing up at one end of the gym. Half the students go to the cone that is tipped over at the other end of the gym. In the middle of the gym, cones are flipped over and others are standing up. On the whistle, students on the cone flip team will turn them up and students on the stand-up team will flip cones over. Use walking, skipping, and running for different rounds.

Workout:

Climb the Mountain. Find a set of stairs outside or in the building. Walk fast up the stairs for 1 minute, slow on the way down.

Activity:

Cone Tag. If you have a cone, you are a tagger. If you get tagged, you must pick up a cone and help the tagging team. The last student without a cone can start a new game. Now if you are tagged, you put your cone down and help taggers.

Activity Focus: Heart Rate

SOCIAL INTERACTION:

Safety during workout; proper etiquette for walking up and down stairs

WEEK 1—DAY 4

ENGAGEMENT IN PHYSICAL ACTIVITY:

Instant Activity:

Have students run in place, and then try to find the pulse and calculate heart rate on wrist. Have them do it before, during, and after running in place.

HEALTH-RELATED FITNESS:

Warm-Up:

Tail Tag. Each student will wear a piece of fabric on his/her hip. They can run around and try to steal other tails. If you get your tail pulled, you are not out. Count how many you have when the game ends.

Workout:

Truth Fitness. All students stand on a line. The teacher makes a statement and if it is true, they will run to the opposite side and back. If it is false, they stay and do jumping jacks. Example—"The world is flat."

Activity:

Triangle Tag. Three players hold hands. The fourth player will try to grab a tail that one player in the group of three has on their hip. The group of three moves in a circle so that the flag cannot be pulled. Give a good demo for triangle tag.

SOCIAL INTERACTION:

Safety Note: Students must stay on feet during all activities.

WEEK 1—DAY 5

ENGAGEMENT IN PHYSICAL ACTIVITY:

Instant Activity:

Walking/Jogging Backward. Obviously, this has some inherent risks, so have the students "social distance" as much as possible as well as staying vocal. Moving backward though is another skill we will all use at some point.

HEALTH-RELATED FITNESS:

Warm-Up:

Cone Flip or Water Bottle Flip. Groups of two with one cone or water bottle in between them. They try to get a cone or bottle to stand after they flip it. If they do, they stay and then do an exercise (e.g., Instant Activity Day 1). If they don't, they have to run to another group and play a new player.

Workout:

Partner Fitness. One partner stands on a line and does an exercise while the other runs back and forth. Keep switching exercise and how many times they run.

Activity:

Cone Stack Relay. Keep the same partners. Run to the end of the area with a cone. Repeat the process while switching back and forth with his/her partner. Have different patterns or stacks that they have to create.

WEEK 2—DAY 1

ENGAGEMENT IN PHYSICAL ACTIVITY:

Instant Activity:

Tape some hopscotch games on the gym floor. Have students move through them until class starts.

HEALTH-RELATED FITNESS:

Warm-Up:

Hopping Around. Teach hopscotch.

Workout:

HIIT (High-Intensity Interval Training) Style Workout. Hop on one foot for 20 seconds and rest for 10 seconds for eight rounds. Keep switching feet. Hop on both for a modification.

Activity:

Muscle Tag. When you are tagged by tagger you must perform an exercise for your biceps or triceps. Have stations around the gym with pictures of exercises. Example: dips, push-ups (full and modified), plank hold, shoulder touches.
    (Yes—these can be hard—but we must raise the bar.)

Activity 2:

> *Crocodile Plank (Animals in Motion)*—Level 1
> "Move slowly through the swamp."
> Maintain push-up plank position with varying challenges.
>
> *Walking Croc*—Level 2
> Alternate lifting hands off floor while planking.

Dancing Croc—Level 3
Alternate lifting hand to opposite shoulder while planking.

BENEFITS OF ACTIVITY:

Weekly Mini Lessons: Muscle strength (avoiding pediatric dynapenia!)

Activity Focus: Components of being physically fit—muscle strength and endurance

WEEK 2—DAY 2

ENGAGEMENT IN PHYSICAL ACTIVITY:

Instant Activity:

Encourage students to dance as they walk in the gym. Play music.

HEALTH-RELATED FITNESS:

Warm-Up:

Freeze Dance. Play some music and freeze it to get students "out." Once out they run around the cones or continue to dance outside of boundaries.

Workout:

Chair Squats Using Chairs or Bleachers. The squat is the most basic of movements/exercises. Most children at this age should be able to do this fairly naturally, though they still may need some coaching to achieve a perfect squat. There is no problem literally allowing them to sit on the bleacher at the bottom of the squat to emphasize this is the position we want them moving into.

Activity:

Relays. Must perform strength exercise before you run, skip, or speed walk to a cone and back. Shuttle Relays, Team Relays, Pass the Baton Relays will work for this activity.

Additional Activity for Leg Strength Exercises:

    Gecko Lunge (Animals in Motion)
    "Camouflage yourself and move slowly"
    Different lunge challenges

Inching Gecko—Level 1
Alternate forward lunge with hands on hips

Strutting Gecko—Level 2
Alternate forward lunge with arm movements

Hiding Gecko—Level 3
Alternate backward lunge

Activity Focus: Leg strength

WEEK 2—DAY 3

ENGAGEMENT IN PHYSICAL ACTIVITY:

Instant Activity:

Have students perform chair/air (not touching seat) squats with a friend until class starts. Practice perfect form!

HEALTH-RELATED FITNESS:

Warm-Up:

Individual Kickball. Students partner up and get two small cones and a soft-style kickball. If you are using a gym, use the sidelines for a basketball court to organize students. One partner stands on one sideline across from his/her partner. Each pair should be an arms-length from the pair next to them. The game starts when partner A pitches to partner B. Partner B kicks the ball anywhere in the gym. Partner A has to go and get the ball and then try to tag or throw the ball at partner B. Partner B is running back and forth between the two cones until partner A gets back with the ball to make the out. Partner A and B switch roles. Partner A is now kicking and partner B is the pitcher. There will be several individual kickball games going on at once. Use music as a stop and go for the game.

Other rules: You may not touch another ball at any point during the game. Base runners must run straight back and forth and stay in their baseline. When throwing the ball at a base runner, it must be done in a respectful way (underhand toss).

Workout:

Perform activities in between cones (bear crawl, crab walk, plank walk).

Bear Crawl (Animal in Motion)
"Grin and bear it."
Hold a bear crawl position.

Bear Creep—Level 1
Move through space in a bear crawl position.

Bear Scuttle—Level 2
Alternate lifting a hand off floor while holding the bear crawl position.

Bear Shuffle—Level 3
Lift opposite hand and foot off floor while holding bear crawl position.

Activity:

Partner Tag. Hold hands with a partner and tag other groups (use partner from kickball game). If you get tagged, hold your partner's feet so they can do four sit-ups and then switch in order to get back in the game.

Activity Focus: Core strength

WEEK 2—DAY 4

ENGAGEMENT IN PHYSICAL ACTIVITY:

Instant Activity:

Have muscle group pictures on cones and see if students can perform a muscle strength exercise for each group (e.g.: quads/legs—chair squats; abdominals—sit-ups).

HEALTH-RELATED FITNESS:

Warm-Up:

Circle Hoop. Place six to eight hula hoops in the center of a circle of students. Students need to stand close to a partner. Flip a coin and if it is heads, the student that decided to represent heads must run around the circle of students. When they return to their partner, they do hand slap, hand slap, foot slap, foot slap and then try to get into an empty hula hoop. Repeat the process and modify as the game progresses (take a hoop away). Students must stay on feet and if a hoop is full, they cannot attempt to get in it.

Workout:

Fitness Stations. Have posters of different activities for Muscle Strength around the area. Students run to each station and perform exercise until music stops. They should try to get to each station a certain number of times. Have pictures of muscle groups that each exercise targets.

Activity:

Two teams—one team on a kicking line shoulder to shoulder and the other spreads out as fielders and one pitcher. Pitchers pitch the ball to one student on the kicking line. The whole kicking team will run from one end of the area to the other. The fielders try to get all three outs from that one kick—by trying to catch the ball on the fly (one out) and tagging opposing players as they run by. If they don't succeed, the kicking team keeps kicking; otherwise they switch.

WEEK 2—DAY 5

ENGAGEMENT IN PHYSICAL ACTIVITY:

Instant Activity:

Introduce Cardio Fitness Race Day.

HEALTH-RELATED FITNESS:

Activity:

Over/Under/Around and Through. Find something to go over, under, around, and through. (How many can you get?)

Workout:

Dynamic Stretching. Show the importance of moving while stretching after a warm-up game.

    This is an important concept they can never learn too soon. You cannot effectively stretch cold muscles. Stretches are much more useful when done to warm tissues.

Activity:

Every Friday is Cardio Race Day!

Purpose—Assess Cardio Fitness and Show Improvement. You can display a bulletin board in your space with improvements or class goals (pitting one class against the other can be motivating).

Cardio Race—Run Around the School or a Selected Loop. Each week the student will have the opportunity to beat his/her personal record as well as trying to improve the class record.

SOCIAL INTERACTION:

Talk about Cardio Fitness Fridays
Goal setting (SMART)

WEEK 3—DAY 1

ENGAGEMENT IN PHYSICAL ACTIVITY:

Instant Activity:

Leave cones around the gym and see how many students can touch while running at different speeds.

HEALTH-RELATED FITNESS:

Warm-Up:

Mailbox Tag. Three taggers will chase students. If they are tagged, they must take a knee and put up a hand. Others can free them when they put mail tag (hand) down.

Workout:

Sprint Track. Students can sprint the track and then walk back using good form. If possible, show some slow motion of Olympic sprinters to see how their arms, head, and torso are involved with good running form.

Activity:

Racetrack Pursuit. Two teams, one on each side of the area. First person in line chases the first from the other line until they catch the person in front of them. The relay continues until you have a winner. Olympian form!

SOCIAL INTERACTION:

Introduce RPE (Rate of Perceived Exertion): A self-reported scale ranging from 1 to 10. A very light activity such as watching TV is a "1"; a max effort all-out sprint would be a "10."

How Do You Feel During a Slow, Moderate, and Fast Activity? We appreciate there are perceived exertion scales that correspond to heart rate—thus 20 would equate to a heart rate of 200 and 6 (a heart rate of 60) would be baseline. This is a bit more complicated and maybe best for the older students.

WEEK 3—DAY 2

ENGAGEMENT IN PHYSICAL ACTIVITY:

Instant Activity:

How many laps (forward or backward) can you get around the gym/area before class starts?

HEALTH-RELATED FITNESS:

Warm-Up:

Team Tag. Make four teams and time them for how long it takes one team to tag the other three teams. Repeat until all four teams have gone.

Workout:

Same sprint track as yesterday but more laps and moderate pace.

Activity:

Pass the Baton Relay. Each member does a lap around the area until all four have gone. Continue discussion about RPE.

WEEK 3—DAY 3

ENGAGEMENT IN PHYSICAL ACTIVITY:

Instant Activity:

How many laps can you get around the gym/area before class starts?

HEALTH-RELATED FITNESS:

Warm-Up:

Extinction Tag. Four teams with different colors (use wrist bands or some-thing to distinguish). If you are tagged by another team, someone from your team has to tag you back into the game. If your team is all tagged out, you must run three laps around the playing area to get back into the game.

Workout:

Same track but now use a slow pace to run for a longer period of time (cardiovascular endurance training).

Activity:

Cardio Kickball. Teacher pitches five balls continuously until the whole kicking line has kicked. The fielders must get the balls back to the teacher so that she/he always has a ball to pitch. If there is no ball there for the teacher to roll, it's a point for the kicking team. After the kicker kicks, they run the three bases. The teams switch after all members have kicked.

WEEK 3—DAY 4

ENGAGEMENT IN PHYSICAL ACTIVITY:

Instant Activity:

How many laps can you get around the gym/area before class starts?

It does not always have to be new. Most youngsters appreciate a certain amount of knowing, of repetition.

HEALTH-RELATED FITNESS:

Warm-Up:

Bowling Tag. Players holding a ball cannot move and are trying to bowl it at other students and hit below their knees. If a student is hit, they must perform an exercise to get back in the game.

Workout:

Race Prep Day. Working through different running paces in prep for *Cardio Friday*!

Activity:

Secret Agent Tag. Students (18–20) form a circle and stand with their eyes closed. Teacher taps two players once on the shoulder, and they are now the taggers (the "bad guy/gal"). The teacher also taps two players twice on the shoulder, and they are now the Secret Agents (helpers). Teacher asks all students to open their eyes and spread out. Teacher may signal or start music to begin play. Students move slowly around the space. The taggers (the "bad guys/gals") will begin tagging players. Once tagged the student must stop and perform an exercise until a Secret Agent can tag them back into the game. The best part about Secret Agent Tag is that no one knows who the taggers (the "bad guys/gals") or Secret Agents are until they are seen tagging or helping.

Variations: If you are tagged by a tagger, you cannot give up their identity. If both Secret Agent taggers are tagged, the game will be over and it's time to start a new round.

Revenge Tag. Every player is a tagger. If you are tagged, you must stop and perform an exercise until the player that tagged you gets tagged. They will now have to sit and perform an exercise and you are back in the game.

Other rules: tag nicely, eyes up when you are running and tagging.

WEEK 3—DAY 5

ENGAGEMENT IN PHYSICAL ACTIVITY:

Instant Activity:

How many laps can you get around the gym/area before class starts? Music playing for Race Day—stickers ready! Make this a fun and engaging road race style day.

HEALTH-RELATED FITNESS:

Warm-Up:

Pre-race Jog

Workout:

Dynamic Stretch. Show the importance of stretching after a warm-up game. Discuss difference from static stretching.

Activity:

Cardio Race Day! Now that they have the idea from last week, we can bump things up. Importantly though, make sure all are successful and thus showing effort. Have a small track that all can get around. Every time they pass the start, they can get a sticker. They should aim to beat sticker count every Friday. The next level might be a small candy treat if they beat their laps from last week. *(That is Dr. O'Neill's idea—he is weak!)*

WEEK 4—DAY 1

ENGAGEMENT IN PHYSICAL ACTIVITY:

Instant Activity:

Have soft objects around the area that students can throw to certain targets.

HEALTH-RELATED FITNESS:

Warm-Up:

Overhead Throw. Students do a soccer-style overhead "throw in" to their partner. Ball size is not terribly important.

Workout:

Upper Body Day. Working on triceps and biceps for throw strength. Push-ups, planks, and dips. Reps 10, 8, 6, 4, 2.

Additional Activities for Upper Body Strength:

> *Mountain Goat Climbers (Animals in Motion)*
> "Quick feet to flee the prowling wolf."

> *Mountain Goat Walk—Level 1*
> Alternate walking knees into chest while mountain climbing.

> *Mountain Goat Jog—Level 2*
> Increase speed of the mountain climber.

> *Mountain Goat Kicks—Level 3*
> Bring foot to opposite hand.

Activity:

Introduce Basic Throwing Cues. Have targets around the area and points for hitting with the object. How many points can you get in 2 minutes? Your partner will coach your throws using cue words. (Eyes at target. Drive with legs. Follow through.)

> *I talk a lot in the book about not taking time from PE to teach skills. That said, throwing is a motion we all use at some point—not just on the athletic field. Keeping your eyes on a target and using your whole body is something we should all learn as it pertains to many everyday movements.*

SOCIAL INTERACTION:

Safety: Clear path for any projectiles.

WEEK 4—DAY 2

ENGAGEMENT IN PHYSICAL ACTIVITY:

Instant Activity:

Have mini-goals (two cones work as well) and balls out for students to kick.

HEALTH-RELATED FITNESS:

Warm-Up:

Partner Kick. Same as day one but kicking.

Workout:

Leg Day to improve kicking form.
Chair squats and lunge. Reps 10, 8, 6, 4, 2.

Activity:

Kick the Can. Play a version of kick the can with a soft ball.

SOCIAL INTERACTION:

Must kick from the cone area.

WEEK 4—DAY 3

ENGAGEMENT IN PHYSICAL ACTIVITY:

Instant Activity:

Have a standing long jump set up for students to challenge themselves. Also, add a vertical jump wall challenge. They can jump and
stick a Post-it or tape to a certain spot on the wall (can put students'
initials on Post-it/tape).

HEALTH-RELATED FITNESS:

Warm-Up:

Partner Jump. Hula hoops on the floor around the area and have students run around and jump in and out, up and down inside of, or side
to side inside of hoops.

Workout:

Tabata. Twenty seconds of work with a 10-second break for eight
rounds. Have students perform different styles of jumping for each 20
seconds of work.
  Tabata can be used with any and every type of exercise.

  Frog Squat (Animals in Motion)
  Different squat challenges.

  Frog Crouch—Level 1
  Perform a squat with thighs parallel to ground and hands on hips.

Frog Jump—Level 2
Perform a squat then jump off the ground swinging arms overhead.

Frog Tuck—Level 3
Perform a squat and jump off the ground tucking knees toward the chest.

Activity:

Hula Hoop Mania. Have students run around and call a number. They must get that many students into a hoop. Leftover students must perform exercises before the next round.

WEEK 4—DAY 4

ENGAGEMENT IN PHYSICAL ACTIVITY:

Instant Activity: Choice

HEALTH-RELATED FITNESS:

Warm-Up:

Partner Run. Review form with your partner while you run around the area.

Workout:

Mountain Climbers and High Knees. Reps 10, 8, 6, 4, 2.

Activity:

Mat Ball. Place three big tumble mats out on the floor in a home plate, first base, and third base position (there is no second base). Make two teams and send one team to home for kicking and the other team to the field for defense. The pitcher pitches a soft kickball to the first kicker and then the second if the first makes it to first base without earning an out. This continues and the game will be played like a regular kickball game, but several students can occupy the bases. You don't have to run until you feel it is strategically safe. The kicking team can run around the bases twice unless an individual earns an out. That individual will return to the kicking line. Play until there are three outs and then switch sides. To earn an out, the fielding team can catch a kicked ball, tag a runner, or make a play to first after a kicker kicks.

WEEK 4—DAY 5

ENGAGEMENT IN PHYSICAL ACTIVITY:

Instant Activity: Choice

HEALTH-RELATED FITNESS:

Warm-Up:

Pre-race Jog

Workout:

Dynamic Stretching. Show the importance of moving while stretching after a warm-up game.

Activity:

Cardio Race Day!!

   Beat your sticker count!!!

   Set a timer and see how many laps students can get—the time can slightly increase each week, but the main goal is to show consistent improvement.

ELEMENTARY CURRICULUM EQUIPMENT (COSTS):

Cones—Rainbow Dome Cones—$55
Popsicle sticks—$9
Pictures of strength activities, dance moves
Stairs
Bleachers or benches
10–12 balls (soft kickball style)—$77
Stickers—$15
Music
Pieces of fabric—foot long to make tails for tail tag—$5
Whistle—$6
Stopwatch—$10
Hula Hoops (8–10)—$45

Middle School Curriculum

ENGAGEMENT IN PHYSICAL ACTIVITY:

Meet CDC guidelines of 60 or more minutes a day of moderate to vigorous intensity aerobic physical activity, and muscle- and bone-strengthening activity at least 3 days a week.

One of the "Western diseases" rarely discussed is osteoporosis. If children do not load their bones, thus stimulating growth before the age of 35 (that is when we stop adding calcium to our bone "bank"), this will be another disease that we will be seeing in epidemic proportions in 50 years.

HEALTH AND SKILL-RELATED FITNESS:

Understand intensity; aerobic versus anaerobic energy systems; know the health-related fitness components; understand physiological responses to physical activity; understand the effect of physical activity on body systems such as heart rate. Each day this is broken down into Warm-Up, Workout, and Activity.

(Please note, some activities are described above in the Elementary Curriculum.)

BENEFITS OF ACTIVITY:

Appreciate the impact of regular physical activity on health (e.g., healthy weight, efficient heart and lungs, enhanced muscle strength and endurance, strong bones, fewer sick days, more energy!).

SOCIAL INTERACTION:

Show respect for people of similar and different skill/fitness levels; encourage peers, engage in respectful communication—refrain from "put-downs."

WEEK 1—DAY 1

ENGAGEMENT IN PHYSICAL ACTIVITY:

Instant Activity:

Use a whiteboard with several pens available. Have students run around and when they need a break write on the board: What is the longest distance or longest amount of time you have run for? Hopefully, they will soon all be running for the entire time before the warm-up starts.

HEALTH-RELATED FITNESS:

Warm-Up:

Tic-Tac-Toe Relays. Tape tic-tac-toe boards on the gym floor. Teams of three compete against other teams of three. Make x's and o's out of paper or cardboard. Students run to place an "x" or "o" in a space until a tic-tac-toe is accomplished.

Workout:

Jump and Jog. Outside activity working on Cardio endurance. Lateral jump 10 reps, run a lap, jump 20 reps, run a lap, jump 30, run a lap . . .

Activity:

Team Tag. Make three or four teams—each team will tag all others for time.

Activity Focus: Cardio endurance

BENEFITS OF ACTIVITY:

Have a bulletin board available for students to add why they believe physical activity is important. (For every joke answer, they need to provide a serious answer.)

   Why PE?

SOCIAL INTERACTION:

Cheer for the team during tic-tac-toe and encourage high fives at the end of games.

WEEK 1—DAY 2

ENGAGEMENT IN PHYSICAL ACTIVITY:

Instant Activity: Choice

HEALTH-RELATED FITNESS:

Warm-Up:

Rock Paper Scissors (RPS) Loop Run. Split students in groups of four and put them in each corner of the gym. When the music plays, students will pick someone to play RPS with. If you win, you run to the next corner. If you lose, you stay and wait to play another player. First student to get six laps should yell "DONE" as loud as possible.

Workout:

Race Track. Half of the students should run around the perimeter and the other half stay in the middle doing an exercise (sit-ups, push-ups, mountain climbers). Race track runners pass as many students as possible.

Activity:

Extinction Tag. Four teams; if you get tagged by another team, only your team can tag you back in the game. If you get tagged, do a plank hold while waiting to be freed by a team member. If your team is out, you must run three laps and do two perfect push-ups together to get back in the game.

Activity Focus: Muscle strength

WEEK 1—DAY 3

ENGAGEMENT IN PHYSICAL ACTIVITY:

Instant Activity:

Five Components of a Physically Fit Person—Worksheet. (Cardiac endurance, Strength, Muscular endurance, Flexibility, Body composition)
     The five components of physical fitness define overall health. These components define how well your body performs in each of the five categories. Understanding them will help to develop exercise plans for individuals. Teaching these during PE class is important and valuable. Students are learning vocabulary that relates to personal and lifelong fitness.

HEALTH-RELATED FITNESS:

Warm-Up:

Revenge Tag

Workout:

Tabata. Twenty seconds of work and 10 seconds of break.
     Round 1—Jumping Jacks; Round 2—Lateral Jumps; Round 3—Planks.

Activity:

Team Pursuit. Relay chase game—think track cycling (YouTube it!). Two teams will line up on opposite sides of the playing area. The first runners start running around a track. They hand off to the next player on their team. This game continues until a player catches up to a player from another team.

WEEK 1—DAY 4

ENGAGEMENT IN PHYSICAL ACTIVITY:

Instant Activity:

Goal setting and/or predicting results for all assessments.

We discussed SMART goal setting for our rebranded PE earlier—simply a takeoff on personal goal setting. This is one of those times where ideally the PE teacher could meet one-on-one with the student and commit goals to writing.

HEALTH-RELATED FITNESS:

Warm-Up:

Pizza Tag. Students hold a frisbee on the palm of one hand. They will move around in a designated space while trying not to drop their pizza (frisbee). The object of this game is for all students to try to knock pizzas off of other students' hands so that they hit the floor. If this happens, the student with the pizza on the floor must pick it up and go to the designated exercise area. A board with different body weight exercises (sit-ups, push-ups, lunges, jumping jacks) can be posted in that area. Students will have to perform an exercise for a certain amount of repetitions before returning to the game.

Other rules: You cannot hold your pizza against your body. You cannot hold your pizza above your head. If your pizza hits the ground at any point, you must go and exercise.

Activity:

Fitness Assessments
    Max sit-up test (1 min)
    Max push-up (1 min) (may modify)
    Step-ups and max line or lateral jumps (1 min)

Activity Focus:
    Five components of fitness
    Value of assessments
    Doing your best
    Goal setting for next assessment

WEEK 1—DAY 5

ENGAGEMENT IN PHYSICAL ACTIVITY:

Instant Activity: Choice

HEALTH-RELATED FITNESS:

Warm-Up:

Tail Tag

Workout:

Dynamic Stretching. Show the importance of moving while stretching after a warm-up game.

    This is an important concept they can never learn too soon. You cannot effectively stretch cold muscles. Stretches are much more useful when done to warm tissues.

Activity:

Mile Run for Time

BENEFITS OF ACTIVITY:

Track progress for all assessments.
Celebrate improvements and personal growth.
Static stretching vs. dynamic stretching overview.

SOCIAL INTERACTION:

Encourage students during fitness testing. Each result is for them to measure improvement for the next set of fitness tests.

WEEK 2—DAY 1

ENGAGEMENT IN PHYSICAL ACTIVITY:

Instant Activity:

Write on whiteboard: 50 sit-ups, one lap; 40 sit-ups, one lap; 30 sit-ups, one lap; 20 sit-ups, one lap; 10 sit-ups, one lap

    Complete as much as possible within Instant Activity time frame.

HEALTH-RELATED FITNESS:

Warm-Up:

Mat Ball. See Elementary Week 4, Day 4, above.

Workout:

Yoga/Flexibility. Basic yoga postures:

- Cat
- Cow
- Downward dog
- Upward dog
- Child's pose
- Warrior

We discussed having local experts come in to supplement the PE lessons. If you are not comfortable demonstrating some basic yoga postures, this would be a great time for that as yogis seem invariably generous with their time. There are also several yoga programs online.

Activity:

Soccer Unit. Dribble Square—all students are taught proper cues for a soccer dribble. Practice using cues in a grid while introducing new concepts along the way—for example, using cut moves or direction changes.

BENEFITS OF ACTIVITY:

Review the five components of being physically fit.
Review assessment scores.

WEEK 2—DAY 2

ENGAGEMENT IN PHYSICAL ACTIVITY:

Instant Activity: Stations for dribble and pass

HEALTH-RELATED FITNESS:

Warm-Up:

Individual Kickball. See Elementary Week 2, Day 3, above.

Workout:

Tabata Tuesday. Twenty seconds of work followed by a 10-second rest for eight rounds.

Plank holds/shoulder touches in a plank for song one.
Jump ropes and running for song two.
Alternate front and side kicks for song three.

Activity:

Passing Square. Teach proper cues for passing the soccer ball using a grid. Advance activity by adding new challenges.

Set up cones and have the students use this smaller area to create passing options. Half of the students will have a ball while the other half is moving around in open space. The students with the ball will be looking to deliver a good pass to any open player. This drill teaches the importance of a good pass as well as teaching students to move around and find open areas to receive a pass. A small field is a great way to keep eyes on all students while they are developing basic soccer skills.

A grid is a smaller version of a soccer field. These can be set up with cones. This is a great way to organize drills and activities. You can make several grids so that every student is participating and involved. It is an easy way to watch all participants while teaching fundamentals.

Cues are great for teaching students new skills. These cues can be used to emphasize consistent and deliberate practice. An example of a cue for a good soccer pass would be a hard pass on the ground—this cue is meaningful and important. It is short and simple and it reminds students that a hard pass will be more effective so that the defense cannot take it away.

BENEFITS OF ACTIVITY:

Muscle Endurance Day. Goal setting for assessments

SOCIAL INTERACTION:

Consider hosting a *World Cup Event:* Invite other "experts" to visit. This is a good time for studying countries, languages, food for sports nutrition, sportsmanship, and music. The list is endless, but it brings in some new voices and community involvement.

WEEK 2—DAY 3

ENGAGEMENT IN PHYSICAL ACTIVITY:

Instant Activity: Choice

HEALTH-RELATED FITNESS:

Warm-Up:

Team Kickball. Focus on cues for kicking.

Workout:

Teams of Four for Push-Ups and Sit-Ups (Muscle Strength Day). First teammate does one with proper form and technique, second teammate does two, third does three, fourth does four, and then back to first teammate who completes five (continue for a certain amount of time or one song). Repeat for sit-ups.

Activity:

Soccer Mini Grid. Games of keep-away or knock-cone-over soccer while focusing on cues for dribble and pass.

SOCIAL INTERACTION:

Celebrate good passes and good soccer decisions with a point system.

WEEK 2—DAY 4

ENGAGEMENT IN PHYSICAL ACTIVITY:

Instant Activity: Choice

HEALTH-RELATED FITNESS:

Warm-Up:

One-Base Kickball. Use a big cone. You must tag cone before ball gets back to pitcher. Focus on kicking form.
  Again, we do not care so much about "kicking." We care about asymmetric motions that require balance. Kicking in karate, kicking a ball, kicking in dance, kicking as you jump across a puddle—all provide similar motor learning.

Workout:

Ladder for Agility and Speed. Motor skill focus

Activity:

Six-Goal Soccer. Three teammates on each side with six different lines at each goal will create a three versus three scenario. Focus on dribble pass and having the option to pass through any of the other teams' three goals. Advance the activity by starting to talk about the first defender and role of defense and offense.

WEEK 2—DAY 5

ENGAGEMENT IN PHYSICAL ACTIVITY:

Tracking mile time
Improvement Club
Goal setting

HEALTH-RELATED FITNESS:

Warm-Up:

Cardio Kickball. The pitcher continuously pitches to the kicking team. All members run around bases. Every time the pitcher reaches down for a ball and there is no ball to pitch it is a point for the kicking team. Fielders must retrieve the balls that have been kicked and get them back to the pitcher.

Workout:

Dynamic Stretching: (completed after heart rate has been increased)

- Toy soldiers: Swing arm around while kicking leg in a toy soldier marching fashion (hamstring and arms)
- Three steps and touch your toes (hamstring)
- Arm circles—small and big (deltoids)
- Three steps and bring heel to backside (quadriceps)
- Three steps and bring toes toward shin (calf)
- High knees
- Kick backside
- Grapevine

Mobility: Use rollers to target muscle groups (kitchen rolling pins work well if rollers are not available)—roll over muscles to get them ready to move.

Use tennis balls, lacrosse balls, or baseballs to roll feet and other parts of the body. Place the ball against the wall to roll back muscles.

Activity:

Mile Run Day

BENEFITS OF ACTIVITY:

Speed, Agility, and Quickness—SAQ
Motor Skills

SOCIAL INTERACTION:

Weekly Mile Cheer Club. Celebrate individual victories.

WEEK 3—DAY 1

ENGAGEMENT IN PHYSICAL ACTIVITY:

Football rules posted. Team names hung around gym. Make squads for fun that represent teams in the NFL and be able to find on the map.

HEALTH-RELATED FITNESS:

Warm-Up:

Focus on throwing cues.

Don't overthink the room here. We say in the book you do not need to learn how to throw a football, just like you do not need to overhead throw a soccer ball, chest pass a basketball, or "shot put" any size ball. That does not mean it is not fun and you are not learning some movement patterns. Mix it up. Let them use their imaginations as long as their whole body is involved launching the projectile!

Workout:

Yoga and Mobility Stations

Activity:

Throwing different objects for distance; if in a large space, run and get it. Throwing at a target. Throwing to a moving target.

Tag Game. Students can walk fast, run, or skip in a designated area. Pick two students to be taggers. They will try to tag as many students as possible. Have two objects (soft-style ball) that can be used by the students who are avoiding being tagged. They can throw the ball around to others who are being chased. If you have the ball, you cannot be tagged.

Other rules: A small space for this game is helpful (how often do you hear that!). The players with the ball can only hold onto it for 10 seconds before giving it to another player. If the tagger tags the player with the ball, that player will become the tagger.

WEEK 3—DAY 2

ENGAGEMENT IN PHYSICAL ACTIVITY:

Instant Activity: Choice

HEALTH-RELATED FITNESS:

Warm-Up:

Pin or Cone Knockdown. Two teams try to knock other teams' cones down while carrying any type (soft) ball. They can travel to the other team's side but can also be tagged. A player must receive a throw from a teammate to get back in the game.

Workout:

Tabata Tuesday
    Push-Ups/Sit-Ups song one
    Mountain Climbers/Core Twists song two
    Focus: Muscle endurance

Activity:

Target-throwing contests, stationary and moving. Use all types of objects. (Though perhaps not axes just yet!)

WEEK 3—DAY 3

ENGAGEMENT IN PHYSICAL ACTIVITY:

Instant Activity: Choice

HEALTH-RELATED FITNESS:

Warm-Up:

Tail Tag. Use some material to have students put on hip. Play a tail tag game. Students try to steal others.

Workout:

Squat Challenge. Spend time reviewing proper form and technique for a squat. Instead of just a bench or a chair, have several tools to encourage good form. For example: a jump rope under the armpits of a student and you hold ends while facing them. This will help to keep their weight on mid foot/heel. Have pictures and cues hung on the wall. Have items around the gym that they must squat down and pick up using proper form. Partner them up and use a coach/athlete approach (baskets are a good item to pick up!).

The challenge is for good form points.

Activity:

Five Pass. Using good throwing cues, make five complete passes with your team. You can move anywhere with the object, and if the other team intercepts or you drop it, it is the other team's turn to make five passes. Use a football or rugby ball toward the end of the game to increase difficulty.

SOCIAL INTERACTION:

Squat partners and coaching tips from partners. How to coach and use advice.

We discussed earlier John Wooden: Here's what you're doing; here's how I want you to do it; here's how you get there.

It is always easier to see poor form on someone else than on yourself (that's why there are mirrors in health clubs and dance studios). The students at this age are ready to do some teaching/coaching of their own. This is an incredibly powerful tool for engagement and learning.

WEEK 3—DAY 4

ENGAGEMENT IN PHYSICAL ACTIVITY:

Instant Activity: Choice

HEALTH-RELATED FITNESS:

Warm-Up:

Capture the Football/Rugby Ball. Encourage good throwing technique and introduce catching cues.

Workout:

Jump Rope Challenge. 1,000 with a partner—split evenly.

Activity:

Three Versus Three Football
   Intro—Center, QB and receiver (switch roles after one play).
   Moderate—add a defender for receiver.
   Advanced—three versus three game with flag pulling and
      rushing rules.

WEEK 3—DAY 5

ENGAGEMENT IN PHYSICAL ACTIVITY:

Instant Activity: Choice

HEALTH-RELATED FITNESS:

Warm-Up:

Capture Football Game: With added rules (flag pulling, making complete passes before running it over line).
   Football and rugby add the element of a crazy-shaped ball, but this does not mean you cannot do some sort of game using a soccer or basketball instead.

Workout:

Dynamic stretches after mobility

Activity:

Mile Run. Cardio day

SOCIAL INTERACTION:

Weekly Mile Partner Cheer

WEEK 4—DAY 1

ENGAGEMENT IN PHYSICAL ACTIVITY:

Instant Activity: Choice
   We have been giving you a "choice" for some of the engagement activities, but unless there is a compelling teaching point or something left over from the day before, get them moving.

HEALTH-RELATED FITNESS:

Warm-Up:

Rock Paper Corner Tag. Split the students into four equal groups. When the music starts, the students in each corner will find someone to play Rock, Paper, Scissors (RPS) against. If the student wins, they can run around to the next corner and find another player to challenge in a game of RPS. If you lose, you must stay and wait for a player coming from another corner to come and play you. The object of this game is to get around the entire square as many times as you can in a certain time or 10 laps—depending on size of playing area.

Other rules: All students must run in the same direction. If you lose three times in a row, go ahead and run. Play fun music!

Workout:

Yoga/Stretching (Flexibility day). You never know what might grab a child's attention and help maintain their physical identity.

Activity:

Basketball Dribble Circle. Teach cues for proper dribble and ball control.

Game: Put a bunch of cones in the middle of space. Make four teams and one at a time each team member has to dribble and pick up a cone. Play a few rounds and continue to stress good dribbling skills

WEEK 4—DAY 2

ENGAGEMENT IN PHYSICAL ACTIVITY:

Instant Activity: Choice

HEALTH-RELATED FITNESS:

Warm-Up:

Relays Using Basketballs. Continuous relays prevent any student from dribbling alone.

Workout:

Tabata Tuesday. Muscle endurance day

Two songs—try mountain climbers, running, jumping jacks, sit-ups, push-ups, V-ups, Russian twists, and other exercises, and throw them in a hat (students can pick exercises out of hat or choose their own—as long as working multiple muscle groups).

Activity:

Knockout Dribble. Each student will have a basketball. While performing good dribbling skills (eyes up, finger pads, protecting the ball, dribble from waist and below), try to knock away other students' basketball. If your ball is knocked away from you, go grab it, perform a designated exercise (jumping jacks, high knees, split jacks, lateral jumps), and then you can rejoin the game.

Passing introduction
Stations for passing

BENEFITS OF ACTIVITY:

Discuss the benefits of HIIT (high-intensity interval training) style workouts.

WEEK 4—DAY 3

ENGAGEMENT IN PHYSICAL ACTIVITY:

Instant Activity: Choice

HEALTH-RELATED FITNESS:

Warm-Up:

Cone Flip Game. Partner up and one cone each. Try to flip the cone so it stands up. If the cone stands up, you stay at the cone and do jumping jacks while your partner runs to find another student to play.

Workout:

Stair Workout. Find your sets of stairs and mix it up for a good 10–15 minute up and down workout.

Activity:

Introduce basketball shooting cues, zone defense, and play three versus three games.

WEEK 4—DAY 4

ENGAGEMENT IN PHYSICAL ACTIVITY:

Instant Activity: Choice

HEALTH-RELATED FITNESS:

Warm-Up:

Individual Capture Game with a partner. Protect a cone from other classmates. One guard and one player that will go out and try to take other team's cones. Switch roles after a fashion.

Workout:

Football Combine: Set up the following activities and have each student rotate through.

40-yard dash—Sprinting ability.
Shuttle run—Set two cones out that the students have to run and grab (30 feet away). They have to run and grab one cone and bring it back to the start line. Next, run to grab the other cone and sprint past the start line with the cone in hand (for time).
Vertical jump—Have students jump up and stick a sticky note (or a piece of tape) with their initials onto the wall.
Standing jump—For measure.
Throw a football to a target—Something on a cone to knock off. Now try a moving target.

Optional: Set up an obstacle course with some tires to run through, cones to run around (slalom style), and then pick up a football and run it past a finish line.

Keep it fun and light.

This would be an excellent activity to have high school students get involved and help organize.

Activity:

Zone Defense
Teach a simple zone with no press.
Play small games of basketball.

WEEK 4—DAY 5

ENGAGEMENT IN PHYSICAL ACTIVITY:

Instant Activity:

Make NBA teams. *(Again, find them on the map and know a fun fact about the city.)*

HEALTH-RELATED FITNESS:

Warm-Up:

Mini-Basketball Championship Tournament

Workout:

Dynamic Stretching and Mile Day. Cardio day

SOCIAL INTERACTION:

Weekly Mile Partner Cheer

High School Curriculum

ENGAGEMENT IN PHYSICAL ACTIVITY:

Analyze characteristics of sport and physical activities that are personally enjoyable, challenging, and fulfilling; differentiate between intrinsic, extrinsic, task, and goal orientations for participation. Begin discussion of "lifelong" activities.

HEALTH AND SKILL-RELATED FITNESS:

Training principles that affect physical fitness; application of principles of training and FITT principle (frequency, intensity, time, and type); physiological responses (energy expenditure, training zone HR, respiratory rate, resting HR). Each day this is broken down into Warm-Up, Workout, and Activity.

BENEFITS OF ACTIVITY:

Evaluate benefits of regular participation on reduction of chronic disease risks; interrelationship of physiological responses and physical, mental/intellectual, emotional, and social benefits.

SOCIAL INTERACTION:

Initiate positive social behaviors associated with physical activity; design strategies for a diverse group of individuals to encourage effective participation; analyze how cultural diversity enriches and challenges health behavior.

WEEK 1—DAY 1

ENGAGEMENT IN PHYSICAL ACTIVITY:

Instant Activity: Choice

HEALTH-RELATED FITNESS:

Warm-Up:

TAG Mania. Three or four different tag games to get heart rate up: Tail, Everyone It, Extinction, or Ball Tag.

Tail tag—each student puts a piece of cloth or jersey "tail" on their hip (tuck it into your shorts or pants on the side of your body). Find a playing area with boundaries. The object of this game is to run around and take other players' "tails" off their hips. At the end of the game you can count and see how many you have. If a player takes another player's tail, they will put it on their hip. You can take all of the tails off of a player's hip at one time. This is a version of tag, but you are stealing tails instead.

Everyone It tag—find a playing area with some boundaries. Everyone will run around and try to tag each other. If you are tagged, perform some sit-ups until the person who tagged you gets tagged. Now you can enter the game again.

Extinction—This is a tagging game. You will have four different teams, and each team wears a different color jersey. Each team will be tagging the other three colors. For example, if you are on the yellow team, you are trying to tag blue, green, and red. If a yellow player is tagged, they must wait in a sitting position until one of their teammates comes along and tags them back into the game. If an entire team is tagged, they are extinct. They must wait until the next game, and they can perform some exercises or stretches while they wait.

Workout:

Yoga/Flexibility. Basic yoga postures:

- Cat
- Cow
- Downward dog
- Upward dog
- Child's pose
- Warrior
- Consult with your local yogi!

Activity:

Volleyball intro
Passing technique
Drills/Stations/Coaching Stations

BENEFITS OF ACTIVITY:

Why PE? Introduce physical identity (write on whiteboard).
        Difference between dynamic and static stretching.
        Physical identity is a complicated subject to bring up in a time-sensitive situation. For sure the students are ready to have this discussion; we just want to respect their space to blow off some energy. Physical identity is something ideally the teacher could discuss on an individual basis while the class is run by the PE assistant.

SOCIAL INTERACTION:

Write down social benefits of playing an organized sport or participating in an activity. Have small slips of paper and writing utensils available for them to write their name and answers on.

WEEK 1—DAY 2

ENGAGEMENT IN PHYSICAL ACTIVITY:

Instant Activity: Choice

HEALTH-RELATED FITNESS:

Warm-Up:

Rock Paper Scissors Corner Relay

Workout:

Tabata Exercise Session. Four songs—student choices

 Anytime there is "choice" it can be student choice—just ensure that it is not always the same student.

Activity:

Volleyball (though any similar ball can be used)

- Passing against wall
- Passing with partner: Pair confident volleyball players with less confident players
- Coach each other
- Skills test for volleyball pass
- Pass back and forth with a partner

SOCIAL INTERACTION:

Students will create workouts—voice and choice important—give a list of exercises and students will pick for their Tabata routine.

WEEK 1—DAY 3

ENGAGEMENT IN PHYSICAL ACTIVITY:

Instant Activity: Choice

 The more choice we can give to this age group, the better the chance of keeping them on board. Yoga is fine, but they still must be in motion!!

HEALTH-RELATED FITNESS:

Warm-Up:

Two Ways to Win

- Pick two teams.
- Split playing area into equal parts.
- On the far endline of each side of the playing area, set up six big cones with tennis balls on top and place a hula hoop with an object in it behind the cones.
- In the middle of the playing area, set out soft-style balls that will be used to knock the tennis balls off of the cones.

Game 1: Have each team try to knock the tennis balls off the other team's cones.

Game 2: Repeat the rules from Game 1, but you can also try to capture the other teams object in the hula hoop.

Game 3: Steal the object in the hula hoop, and then knock the other team's tennis balls off the cones.

If you are going over to the other team's side, you can be tagged. To get back in the game, you will go to the designated exercise area and perform a set of exercises before returning to the game.

Other rules: You cannot throw the balls at other players. You must tag them. You cannot guard tennis balls for each game. You must play all positions.

Workout:

Squat Day. Review proper form and technique. Partner workout—coaching each other while completing. AMRAP (as many rounds as possible)—10 squats and 10 step-ups—you will take turns so that partner will coach form. Set clock for 10 minutes.

Activity:

Groups of four working on volleyball passing drills. Review form and technique. Every drop ball can result in 10 jumping jacks for a contest at the end of lesson.

BENEFITS OF ACTIVITY:

Muscle Strength. More complicated anatomy introduced (e.g., agonist and antagonist muscles).

WEEK 1—DAY 4

ENGAGEMENT IN PHYSICAL ACTIVITY:

Instant Activity: Choice

HEALTH-RELATED FITNESS:

Warm-Up:

Pin or Cone Knockdown. Two teams try to knock other team's cones down. They can travel to the other team's side carrying any type of ball, but can also be tagged. Must receive a throw from a teammate to get back in the game. Focus on throwing form.

Workout:

Jump Rope. Jump with two feet, jump with one foot, Double Unders (rope rotates under feet two times per jump)—skill work for 3–5 minutes.

Complete for time: 100 jump ropes, 10 sit-ups, 90 jump ropes, 10 sit-ups, 80 jump ropes, 10 sit-ups, 70, 10, 60, 10, 50, 10, 40, 10, 30, 10, 20, 10, 10, 10.

Jumping rope is another one of those activities that has crossover with so many movement patterns that lead to health and safety.

Activity:

Passing V-Ball Over a Net or Line. Partner will give an underhand toss, and other partner must pass the ball to the target or to a designated area.

Play mini two versus two V-ball games.

WEEK 1—DAY 5

ENGAGEMENT IN PHYSICAL ACTIVITY:

Create a Journal for 5K Success. Include nutrition, sleep, distractions to avoid (e.g., video games), starting point, and goals.

HEALTH-RELATED FITNESS:

Warm-Up:

Dynamic Stretching

Activity:

Time a Mile Run. Building a training log for a 5K

BENEFITS OF ACTIVITY:

List benefits of cardio endurance training.

SOCIAL INTERACTION:

Make teams for 5K challenge.

Find a local 5K or create one.

This day spends more time talking, thinking, and planning than most, but with luck we are building some excitement for the 5K. (And they still ran a timed mile!)

WEEK 2—DAY 1

ENGAGEMENT IN PHYSICAL ACTIVITY:

Volleyball Rules clinic. Beach volleyball too!
     This should be on whiteboard ahead of time, and each student can get a handout. It does not have to consume a lot of time. Beach volleyball has become a huge city game. Explore where in your area there are public courts.

HEALTH-RELATED FITNESS:

Warm-Up:

Kick and Run

Workout:

Yoga/Flexibility

Activity:

Introduction to Volleyball Setting and Serving

- Stations for cues
- Serving to a target
- Setting into a basketball hoop
- Small games over a net or a line

BENEFITS OF ACTIVITY:

Anatomy Review: Bones and Muscles.
     Can start introducing things they might hear about in the media: achilles tendon, IT band, scoliosis, stress fractures, and so on. Ask class for ailments they incurred to start discussion.

WEEK 2—DAY 2

ENGAGEMENT IN PHYSICAL ACTIVITY:

Instant Activity: Choice

HEALTH-RELATED FITNESS:

Warm-Up:

Kick and Steal. This game is Mat Ball with a twist. (See Mat Ball rules above.)

Place four cones with a tennis ball or a ring on each cone. For this game, you will add a second and "fourth" base (total of five bases including home). If someone from the kicking team is on second, third, or fourth base, they can try to steal a tennis ball or ring off of the cones that are behind those bases. They must run the stolen object directly to home base. The fielders must use the game ball to tag them or throw underhand at them to get them out. Players who do not choose to go off a base will run the bases in order.

Other rules: Use three outs and then switch fielders and kickers.

Stealing an object is worth three points. Students who score after running bases in order will get one point (you do not round bases twice like Mat Ball).

Workout:

Tabata. Four songs with student choice activities

Activity:

Three Versus Six Volleyball. Working on cues for passing, setting.

Volleyball is a tough skill to master but reacting to something coming at you and if nothing else, having the eye-to-hand coordination to swat it away, is an important life skill. Keep a close eye to notice any students who might struggle with this. No broken glasses!

WEEK 2—DAY 3

ENGAGEMENT IN PHYSICAL ACTIVITY:

Instant Activity: Choice

HEALTH-RELATED FITNESS:

Warm-Up:

Four Square Games. Make rules and courts with the help of students.

Workout:

Pull-Ups and Push-Ups. Introduce banded pull-ups and jumping pull-ups for modifications.

Deck of cards for help with workout—each card symbol can represent a different style of push-up—examples: wide, narrow, tricep.

Everyone who graduates from your school should be able to do some proper push-ups and hopefully at least one pull-up. This is the equivalent of graduating with a sixth-grade reading level.

Activity:

Serve and Retrieve. Go over cues for serving. Overhand or underhand are fine. Play a game of volleyball. Get ready for a tournament.

BENEFITS OF ACTIVITY:

Name muscle groups used during the workout.

WEEK 2—DAY 4

ENGAGEMENT IN PHYSICAL ACTIVITY:

Instant Activity: Choice

HEALTH-RELATED FITNESS:

Warm-Up:

Four Corner Capture Game

Workout:

Speed Workout. Sprints—200 yards (meters) with 20 mountain climbers in between. One-minute rest between each round. FOUR ROUNDS.

Activity:

King of the Court Volleyball Tournament
    People should be pretty gassed from the speed workout. Play it by ear with the volleyball—maybe just a cool-down with some yoga.

WEEK 2—DAY 5

ENGAGEMENT IN PHYSICAL ACTIVITY:

Journal work—5K goal setting.
    Putting things in writing is a powerful tool in goal setting. For any goal. Let them know these are life skills—not just something for PE.

HEALTH-RELATED FITNESS:

Warm-Up:

Ultimate Frisbee Game

Workout:

5K Prep
>   Run 2×800 for time
>   Work with team
>   Review journal

BENEFITS OF ACTIVITY:

Heart rate review—target, max, etc.

WEEK 3—DAY 1

ENGAGEMENT IN PHYSICAL ACTIVITY:

Importance of flexibility and mobility when training for a 5K.
When talking about things that most teens might not think about regarding health such as flexibility, it is never a bad time to again emphasize sleep and proper nutrition. How many hours did you sleep last night? What did you have for breakfast this morning?

HEALTH-RELATED FITNESS:

Warm-Up:

Individual Kickball

Workout:

Yoga. Flexibility day

Activity:

Basketball Drills and Stations

BENEFITS OF ACTIVITY:

Using sport as a workout in life after school
>   *Muscle Soreness:* how to treat and recover

WEEK 3—DAY 2

ENGAGEMENT IN PHYSICAL ACTIVITY:

Instant Activity: Choice

HEALTH-RELATED FITNESS:

Warm-Up:

Pizza Tag. See Middle School Week 1, Day 4.

Workout:

Tabata Day. Students create their own workout for four songs. Focus on muscle endurance and weaknesses (ask them to identify these and suggest to them solutions).

Activity:

Basketball Shooting Drills. Review cues. Relays for dribble and passing.

WEEK 3—DAY 3

ENGAGEMENT IN PHYSICAL ACTIVITY:

Instant Activity: Choice

HEALTH-RELATED FITNESS:

Warm-Up:

Rock Paper Scissors Relay. Two teams face each other. One at a time, each team comes out and plays RPS. If you win, you advance toward the other team. If you lose, go back to team and the next member comes out to play. The object is to touch the other team's cone first.

Workout:

Squat/Lunge Day. AMRAP—10 squats and 30 walking lunges. Set a time limit.

Activity:

Two versus two basketball games

WEEK 3—DAY 4

ENGAGEMENT IN PHYSICAL ACTIVITY:

Instant Activity: Choice

HEALTH-RELATED FITNESS:

Warm-Up:

Capture Game. Four corners with four of the same colored objects. You must get one of each of the other team's objects to win. If you are tagged, go back to your side.

Workout:

Speed Workout. 2×400s—work with 5K team. Research relation to mile time and pace.

The 400-meter race is the longest "sprint" and thus by definition HURTS! This is why two 400s are almost the equivalent of two 800s in terms of effort. They will need a lot of high fives by the end.

Activity:

Five Versus Five Basketball Games. Modify game to fit each group. Use defense styles to help. Referee picked for each game—review rules.

Again, you might not get to the hoop games. That's OK. Everyone needs to be yelling for the runners.

WEEK 3—DAY 5

ENGAGEMENT IN PHYSICAL ACTIVITY:

Journal work: nutrition and sleep.
Recovery and how to never regret a workout (see yesterday!).
Motivation—intrinsic and extrinsic.
Intrinsic motivation gets back to our mantra of *"Our school is in motion."*
We *want* to be moving because that's what we are born to do.

HEALTH RELATED FITNESS:

Warm-Up: Choice

Workout:

Cardio Day. 5K day. Have students create a course around campus to complete for time. Work with your team.

    This was a big two-day block. Explain that and congratulate! Saturday should be a light activity, adaptation/recovery day. As noted above, this is an excellent time to introduce these concepts.

WEEK 4—DAY 1

ENGAGEMENT IN PHYSICAL ACTIVITY:

Instant Activity: Choice

HEALTH-RELATED FITNESS:

Warm-Up:

Mat Ball

Workout:

Yoga/Flexibility

- Banded exercises for injury prevention
- Bridges
- Monster walks—toes point ahead, squat to half of your height and take large slow steps (with or without band)
- Skater walks—same exercise but bring foot to middle and then back out when stepping (with or without band)
- Lateral walks—face wall and use same slow step pattern. (Perform at a slow pace, keep tension on band around ankles if using one.)

Activity:

Basketball Tournament Bracket Setup
    Hoop practice
    Establish coach and referee for each game.

BENEFITS OF ACTIVITY:

Injury Prevention. Proper footwear for 5K. How did everyone do? Any blisters Saturday?

WEEK 4—DAY 2

ENGAGEMENT IN PHYSICAL ACTIVITY:

Instant Activity: Choice

HEALTH-RELATED FITNESS:

Warm-Up:

Line Basketball. Call number and they come out to court to play.

Workout:

Tabata Day. Students pick exercises—four songs.

Activity:

Basketball Tournament: Make sure less aggressive students have fun and play a role. Games begin!

WEEK 4—DAY 3

ENGAGEMENT IN PHYSICAL ACTIVITY:

Instant Activity: Choice

HEALTH-RELATED FITNESS:

Warm-Up:

No-dribble basketball games using different objects (can use imagination), three steps with object allowed and then pass to teammates.

Workout:

Step-ups, jump squats, jump lunge, and jumping jacks: 50, 40, 30, 20, 10 of each
    Set a time cap and do as much of the workout as you can to leave time for hoops.

Activity:

Basketball Tournament (continued)

WEEK 4—DAY 4

ENGAGEMENT IN PHYSICAL ACTIVITY:

Journal work. Work with team. Organize details for participation in a local 5K.

HEALTH-RELATED FITNESS:

Warm-Up:

Tic-Tac-Toe. Two teams compete against each other and have to run to a large tic-tac-toe board and play until there is a winner.

Workout:

Speed/Track Workout. Two 40s, three 100s, four 200s, and end with two laps at 50% of mile pace.

The instructor can impress upon students that these are serious workouts. If they can complete these with any gas in the tank, they are truly fit. When training for a longer race such as 5K, speed work is part of it (muscle qualities!).

Activity:

Tournament Decided. Have a fun ceremony at the end.

WEEK 5—DAY 5

ENGAGEMENT IN PHYSICAL ACTIVITY:

Organize details for participation in a local 5K.

HEALTH-RELATED FITNESS:

Warm-Up:

Practice a race day *warm-up* for 5K.

Concept that warm-up, stretch, cool down part of exercise and injury prevention

Workout:

Finish basketball tournament and if any remaining time, ask students what they want to do.

MIDDLE SCHOOL/HIGH SCHOOL
CURRICULUM EQUIPMENT NEEDS (COSTS)

Timer watch: $10
Basketballs: six-pack for $75
Soccer balls: six-pack for $80
Volleyballs: six-pack for $80
Cones: $50
Frisbees: $12 each
Miscellaneous balls: 20-plus pack for $80

THE REVOLUTION STARTS NOW
(AND WILL BE TELEVISED!)

You just read an example of what a rebranded PE program should look like. Now it's time to bring it to your school.

The concept of political action is not something that is a natural fit for most of us. I come from New Hampshire where we are known for our grassroots style of governing. Besides having the "First in the Nation" primary for presidential elections, we also have yearly town meetings where citizens can air their thoughts and ideas. At the state level, we have the largest (all-volunteer!) state legislature in the United States, giving us essentially one representative in our capital of Concord for every 2,000 citizens. People in New Hampshire know the importance of having a voice at the federal, state, and local levels and know how to use their own voice in the community and on school boards. But remember, *you have more power than you think.* Just because getting involved may not be the norm where you live, this does not mean you cannot get things done.

How many people are showing up to your school board or town meetings? I am guessing, unless there is a hot button issue, not many. This is where you come in. With limited numbers attending these gatherings, if you are present with energy, urgency, and intention, your voice can have a colossal influence. As a teacher, administrator, health care provider, or even insurance person, you are coming to the meetings with solid credentials. As a parent, having a few others in your corner before launching that first salvo could really tip the scales in your children's favor.

I will spare you the acorn or first step of a journey metaphors but would proffer that the start of a proper revolution can begin with a cup of coffee. The concept of making changes to the school curriculum is significant and for most folks, absolutely terrifying. Most of your peers have grown up with the same limited, sports-oriented PE system, and simply do not know anything else. The world has changed, but PE has not. Yes, the new buzz phrase is moderate to vigorous physical activity (MVPA), but data shows this is simply not happening for a full PE period. So start the way you might start anything—casually asking colleagues, friends, school board members, and parents their opinions in the teachers' room, the school parking lot, outside the grocery store, or at a ballgame (there's some irony!) (P.S. Ask the person whose child is on the bench!). Those who have children that are already on the road to poor health and spending time on video games should be especially interested. For those who show even minimal interest, set up the "hot beverage meeting" and make your case in more detail with what you have learned in this book. Educate them about the importance of this issue. Sadly, if their child is obese now, they are probably never going to recover. Convince them to help carry the load. Getting this topic on the agenda with your PTA or PTO (Parent-Teacher Association or Organization) could also be an option (and perhaps save you from buying anyone tea). Depending on where you live, this group can be very influential, and at the end of the day, revolution is about finding like minds and then creating momentum.

Having a number of people come with you to the school board meeting would be brilliant, but short of that you should at least say "I have spoken to other parents who support this." This statement should go a long way in establishing credibility. If you are super-motivated, you could even bring a petition signed by multiple interested parties. You do not need an army at this point. The folks on the school board are all aware of our children's health crisis; they simply lack the urgency, intention, and knowledge to come up with a solution. You are bringing them an answer having already done the heavy lifting.

The concerns at school board meetings are always the same. The budget, teacher salaries and benefits, the curriculum, the budget, student safety, class size, the budget, and student achievement are some of the more common topics. (Did I mention the budget?) What if you stood up and said that you have a suggestion to improve student achievement that would not affect said budget (remember: It is *always* about the money)? You would be able to hear a pin drop. That's when you mention a recent *USA Today* article about childhood obesity (they seem to have one every few weeks), this book, or drop the name of your pediatrician who was just lamenting how many of her patients lack fitness (this is done every day, by every doctor). Once those words are out you have it: the beginning of a revolution.

Another option is the "key person" strategy. Once you have recognized a few kindred spirits among your colleagues and parents, another avenue is to find someone in a position of influence at the school (it may even be you!). This person does not have to be a PE teacher, but could be an administrator, an athletic director, a coach, a health care provider, or even a classroom teacher willing to take up the cause. When I started this process in my own community, it was more of an uphill battle than even I expected. Despite being able to cite the literature and knowing many potential key people on a personal basis, the inertia was palpable. Everyone was very "interested," and those in the know acknowledged the lack of PE is a huge problem that we need to do something about. Then came the "however": "However, we don't have the time, money, space, or faculty (or interest!) to make the kind of changes you describe."

Or this one: "Doctor, we are not going to legislate our way out of this problem." (And thanks for coming by!)

Let me be clear: I have no real experience convincing people to come over to my way of thinking. As a doctor, people rarely question my counsel, understanding I went to school for many years and have their best interests in mind. What I have as a doctor, and what we all have in this potential PE revolution, is data. We have solid evidence regarding the health crisis in this country as well as science supporting the physical and academic value of a rebranded PE program. Perhaps most importantly, no one is offering any better solution, except asking students to make changes in their lives they are not motivated to make (e.g., "Just say no"). *Maintaining physical identity means you as a parent do not need to motivate children toward healthy behavior—they will automatically make healthier choices.* This, to my mind, is the most effective element of persuasion as we start this revolution. You are not asking for something ethereal or controversial or negative. You are asking to enact something that is recommended by experts all over the world, including, in all likelihood, your own state via its standards for PE. This change will potentially show huge health gains for our next generation, and not (NOT!) if done correctly, cost taxpayers more money.

Using your best Nelson Mandela diplomat voice, ask for example, your superintendent, if he or she is aware of the literature supporting daily PE and its effect on academics and health. Ask how your school district might be acting on this information. Want to be horrified? Ask how much PE the students are getting at every grade level (remember—your children will be in high school at some point, so ask how it works all 13 years). Ask what they are doing in gym class. Are they moving or learning "skills"? (My suggestion would be to not ask at this point about the money, but of course that conversation must come.) Ask these questions because, while 50 years ago they might not have seemed important, in the 21st century they could be key to a happy and healthy life for your son or daughter.

Another thing I have learned the hard way in my life is sometimes one must go "over the head" of the local authorities to get something done. You must be a bit careful here, as ultimately, we want everyone pulling in the same direction. If there is no response at the district level, it might focus them if they receive a letter from someone above them: the state board, county administrator, secretary of education, or governor (assuming these folks respond to your entreaties).

Although it is a difficult task we have before us, we have a lot going in our favor. First, we have history on our side. The importance of physical activity and its connection to learning has been recognized for decades. Although it just seemed to benefit the students and made sense to the teachers in the past, we now have lots of modern science to support our views.

Second, we have little choice. I appreciate the myriad issues confronting our earth and our society. I realize the oceans are full of plastic, that gender and racial inequality continues to be rampant, that another pandemic might be lurking, or that there are children going to bed feeling unsafe. Of course, these are huge problems and must be addressed, but regarding childhood obesity, as individuals we can actually *do* something about it relatively quickly and cheaply. But to start, we must fight the inertia of a 100-year-old PE system that makes little sense today. I also appreciate that some people will not share your views, despite the science. Trust me, however, there are plenty of people in your school district who will come over to your way of thinking. All you need is to get these folks out of the woodwork. No parent wants their child to be inactive, overweight, depressed, and harboring diabetes.

On a less optimistic note (!), did I mention this cause will make you insanely unpopular within certain circles? Right now, the "sports as PE" system is working for a minority of students. Some people will be upset with you thinking that if high school sports are not funded with taxpayer money, their child might miss out on a college scholarship. Well, I have news for them. First, their youngster was probably not getting a scholarship (though perhaps best not to mention that right away!). The percentage of high school students getting a college scholarship for sports is in the single digits. Second, most are partial scholarships, and if parents saved the money they spent on all those travel teams (with youth sports today not uncommonly going to different *countries* for competitions), they would far exceed what they receive in scholarship dollars. Third, if their child is a good enough athlete, they will be discovered in the community club sports and still get their financial aid. And fourth, the child probably did not need that scholarship if they were already going to college. Let me explain.

Athletic scholarships should go to students who, without one, would be closed out of this next level of education. But are most scholarship recipients truly students that would not be otherwise going to college? In other words, were these families not in a financial position to send their child to a community or state institution without this aid? Now, these questions are not considering the sometimes revenue-producing sports of men's basketball and football. Those two sports are outliers and the topics of a huge amount of discussion regarding whether the athletes should be paid, how much time they should be expected to dedicate to their sport, what majors they are allowed to enroll in, and a host of other contentious issues. What I looked at were the "suburban" sports of soccer, field hockey, lacrosse and baseball. My research looked at the zip codes of the hometowns of multiple athletes from multiple schools. Guess what? A majority of the college athletes were from zip codes above the median income level in the United States. I am not saying these families did not appreciate the monetary support the athletic scholarship gave them. I am saying these students most likely come from families that already had the means to send them to a state school without this money.

THINK GLOBALLY, ACT LOCALLY

You will no doubt run into some roadblocks as you attempt to nudge your school district to acknowledge our new reality. Certainly, I did. I found many kindred souls, but it was the rare person who seemed

willing to put their shoulder behind substantial change. Every educator I spoke with was well aware of the problem; however, they seemed
to feel they were powerless to act, despite all the evidence and the fact
that it was working in other places. I finally made progress when an
enlightened superintendent told me she had the "world's greatest gym
teacher" working in her district. This encouraged me to host a roundtable discussion at a local pub. I invited a breadth of folks including
doctors, educators, and business owners. Perhaps not surprisingly, despite providing refreshments, numerous people I invited found reasons to not be there. Many of these were "key people" who I have
known for years. Maybe it was bad timing on that winter night, or
maybe they did not want to rock the boat. (The district many of these
nonattendees were from might be an example of where you need
one of the "above the head" strategies discussed above.) Ultimately,
two principals, one PE teacher and one paraprofessional who often
works in PE, the superintendent and her husband, and one classroom
teacher shot around ideas for 2 hours as I furiously took notes. The
earth did not reverse spin on its axis, but we had a beginning.

   After several meetings following the roundtable, I was able to develop a plan involving Liz Savage (author of the program above) and
one of the principals who attended to organize a pilot project. We established an activity program where 10–20 kids (in a class of 100) came
to school a half hour early every morning for 30 minutes of exercise.
We monitored the academic performance of the children compared to
the same time in previous years, and while not a scientific study, the
results were significant, especially if you ask the teachers in the first
three periods. The active students were more awake, excited, and ready
to learn. Then we asked the parents. They reported their children are
more academically motivated, less antsy at the end of the day, and even
sleeping better. And this should not be surprising as we did not discover
anything new. I have given examples showing the success of schools
that do have a daily PE policy. Knowing the data, why hasn't every
school adopted this policy? My sense is unless you can show it with *your*
children, in *your* hometown, people will just not be ready for change.

MISSION STATEMENT (REPRISE)

We touched on the concept of the mission statement at the end of
the last chapter. A mission statement may not sound crucial to the

function of an organization, yet it can contain the vital elements of what makes something a success or failure. These statements might seem like just words on a page at the front of the school manual that everyone skips over, or on a plaque in the lobby. But a good mission statement can be more than that. It should distill what an institution is about in just a few words and, on a bad day, can have the power to focus our attention on important issues. Mission statements are most important in difficult times. As I write this book, the United States is in the throes of a school shooting epidemic. As solutions are discussed for this heartbreaking problem, understanding what the mission of the school is, what it represents, and what it is supposed to be doing for our children should help guide us toward answers. This is when a properly worded mission statement does its job.

Here again is my example of a potential mission statement. It tries to account for the physical, academic, personal, and societal needs of all students.

Mission Statement

It is our mission at _____ School to provide a safe environment to nurture both the physical and cognitive aspects of our children's lives. When students leave here, they will be happy, fit, and intellectually curious. They will have the education and the desire to be caring citizens of the world, ready to work for the greater good.

I repeat the concept of the mission statement in this section for a specific purpose. Our schools represent many things, far beyond teaching the "3 R's." They are places of growth for all aspects of our students. In addition to the mind and body, these buildings are where the actual glories of childhood take place. Yes, there might be plenty of sorrow and difficulty, but mostly there should be an experience of safety, caring, wonder, and friendship that continues into adulthood. School is a place where children are loved and accepted for who they are and who they might become. Of course, schools are not just for the students. They can be a source of community pride and civic activism. They can be a place of congregation for meetings and voting. At schools, adults make decisions that directly affect the coming generation, who will then inherit the same decisionmaking powers. This is why the mission statement is so important. What is supposed to be happening at schools? Are we charged with raising the next generation of bright, healthy citizens, or is our mission to provide colleges with star athletes? Is our job to graduate healthy humans free of disease, or are we content to send sick children into the world? It is up to you to agitate for your youngsters. Let's look at another strategy: putting pen to paper.

LETTERS FROM THE FRONT

Letter writing might sound a bit old-fashioned, but it is still an excellent way to lay out your argument elegantly and efficiently. A letter will allow you to reach people with whom you are not always able to meet in person—people of influence, such as the superintendent or local politicians. Plus, a physical letter is much harder to ignore (or delete) than an email.

Below are a few examples of letters I encourage you to download and send to your own decisionmakers. These letters and other information can be accessed at *SurvivaloftheFit.net*.

Letter to the School District Superintendent

Dear _____,

Allow me to introduce myself. My name is _____ and I have been living here in _____ for ____ years, with two children at _____ School. First let me say I appreciate the hard work that you and your wonderful staff do on a daily basis for the education of our children. I do, however, have one significant concern.

It has been brought to my attention that physical education classes seem to be less and less of an emphasis as the school day becomes crowded with multiple activities in addition to regular classwork. While I do not envy you and the people who must make the difficult decisions of what goes on the daily schedule, one subject that we know affects all other learning is PE. In his recent book *Survival of the Fit,* Dr. Daniel O'Neill makes a compelling argument of why, without proper activity, not only will students not be physically fit, but it will be harder for them to be mentally fit. Numerous studies have supported this idea and the data would appear irrefutable. In 2019, a study linked physical activity to higher math and spelling scores (Szabo-Reed et al., 2019). In 2017, a meta-analysis of 26 studies including over 10,000 students came to similar conclusions (Álvarez-Bueno et al., 2017).

The "poster child" for this change has been the town of Naperville, Illinois, where they have made PE mandatory for every child, every day. This school district, which was decidedly average 25 years ago, is now in the top 5% of schools in the state for academics and has a miniscule 5% obesity rate compared to the national rate of 20%. In fact, physical activity has been shown in dozens of studies to activate the brain, allowing it to accept all other forms of input, including such topics as math and English. Without a level of fitness, the brain simply cannot accept new knowledge efficiently. In other words, we cannot have STEM without first having fitness!

I have broached this subject with many other parents who are of the same mind. I would very much like to discuss this topic with you further.

Thank you for your attention to this matter. Our school personnel work so hard to educate our children. Giving these youngsters daily, aggressive PE in all grades would seem to be "low hanging fruit" to make their jobs easier and to advance the physical and mental health of the district's students. I look forward to further communication on this subject.

Very truly yours,

Letter to the Governor

Dear Governor _____,

Thank you for taking time from your busy schedule to give attention to this matter.

I am a citizen of _____ served by school district _____. Along with some of my fellow citizens, we are campaigning for more physical education time in our schools. The data on the benefits of daily physical activity for all children in all grades is clear, yet the trend seems to be to offer less physical education (PE), falling well short of the daily need and in fact, national guidelines. The data is irrefutable. In 2019, a study linked physical activity to higher math and spelling scores (Szabo-Reed et al., 2019). In 2017, a meta-analysis of 26 studies including over 10,000 students came to similar conclusions (Álvarez-Bueno et al., 2017). The "poster child" for this change has been the town of Naperville, Illinois, where they have made PE mandatory for every child, every day. This school district, which was near the average 25 years ago, is now in the top 5% of schools in the state for academics and has a miniscule 5% obesity rate compared to the national rate of 20%. In fact, our own state standards (see attached) endorse this concept of daily exercise on both the physical and cognitive aspects of overall health.

(Warning to my letter writers: Most state standards are on board with this concept. If your state is one of the few that does not discuss this issue in detail, you might use another state example, such as Illinois.)

Unfortunately, on the local level, daily PE is not being offered. Others and I have been in touch with our school board, superintendent, principals, and PE teachers. Perhaps due to the "too many cooks" theory, changes are not being enacted. As a result, we now turn to you, Governor _____, for your influence.

The need for daily exercise in all humans, not just children, is one of the few topics where there is no controversy. There is an obesity and health crisis in our country's youth. We have the means and the knowledge to alleviate this; we simply need the will to make changes. We all must realize the life of children today, with processed food and video games, is vastly different than most of our own experiences. You have the power to create a cultural change that could benefit millions. We are also asking for the appointment of a state PE czar to assist the transition to this rebranded PE program.

Thank you in advance for your attention to this matter. For more information, I would point you to Daniel Fulham O'Neill, MD, EdD, and his book on this subject, *Survival of the Fit*. It is a quick read but gets to the heart of this incredibly important subject and how we can achieve results with no significant increase in the education budget. I look forward to your response and input. Please do not hesitate to call if I can be of any further help to move this matter ahead.

Very truly yours,

cc: The Secretary of Education

Letter to PE Teachers

Dear _____,

I hope this finds you well.

My name is _____ and my child is _____. I have been reading about the importance of PE, not just for children's physical fitness, but also for academic achievement. You might be interested in a recent book on the subject, *Survival of the Fit*. In it the author, a sports medicine doctor and sport psychologist, makes a case for PE to be considered the most important link in our child's education since without activity, not only do the muscles atrophy, but the brain suffers as well.

I was curious not only about the amount of PE the students are getting, but also the specific activities students participate in during PE class. From all reports, we are falling far short of the national standard calling for 30–45 daily minutes of *high energy* PE for every student. What can I and my fellow parents and citizens do to help you make this happen? We know the education you received to achieve your PE degree cuts a broad swath. How can we use your knowledge to its maximum advantage? Hiring a paraprofessional assistant? Different equipment/resources? Space? Time?

With a health epidemic gripping this country, and the coming generation poised to have a shorter lifespan than the last, we must do everything in our power to make a difference. Let me help you bring _____ School to the forefront of not just physical education, but all aspects of learning. I look forward to hearing from you.

Very truly yours,

cc: Principal _____

One of the things I have noticed over the decades is the onus for essentially all children's issues disproportionately landing on the schools (educators: Insert "duhh" here.). We need the involvement of everyone in our revolution, and without the dedication of the parents it will not be effective. The parents might be unhealthy, but that does not mean their children need to be. The concepts presented in this book, just like sustainable environmental policies, must be part of the education of parents and students, and must be emphasized each and every day, whenever and wherever possible. This next letter speaks to that concept.

Letter to Parents

Dear Parents,

We hope you are as excited for the upcoming school year as we are. We would like to ask for your help in a new initiative we are introducing in September. The evidence regarding the importance of physical fitness and how it relates to learning is crystal clear. Children who have poor physical fitness will have a harder time learning. In other words, health and fitness are directly related to academic success. Toward that end, we are trying to encourage our students to be moving throughout the school day, especially in the minutes they might have after arriving at school, in gym class, and at recess. In fact, our new mantra is *"Our school is in motion."* We also hope to introduce short periods of exercise at the beginning of many classes.

You can help us, and thus your child, by supporting this new initiative. The healthier the child is coming to school, the better they will do in school. That means making sure they get plenty of outdoor play after school, limit screen time and processed foods, and have fruit and vegetables available at every meal.

The mind and body are truly connected. Thank you for your support as we continue to try to give your child the best education possible.

Very truly yours,

_____'s homeroom teacher

And one more letter from the classroom teachers:

Letter to the School Board

Dear School Board Members,

Education is truly a moving target. This makes things exciting yet also challenging as the world evolves and new scientific research becomes available. In this case, I would like to make you aware of the changing face of children's activity. One change might be obvious: Children rarely play outside after school but commonly stay inside and engage with video games or other time in front of screens. The other change is the overwhelming evidence that activity (play) is directly related to academic success. If a child is coming to school with poor fitness due to bad nutritional choices, obesity, and lack of activity, they will not be ready to learn, no matter the skills and time offered by their teachers.

Toward this end we are asking the school board for two things. First, a reallocation of funds from interscholastic sports teams to PE (unless there are available funds from a different source). This will support the hiring of PE paraprofessionals (teaching assistants) and possibly the purchase of some other needed equipment upgrades (see detailed plan attached*). Second, we ask for your support regarding community relations, impressing on families and alumni the dire need to make these changes regarding the future health of our children.

The world has changed dramatically in the last 50 years, and the medical and educational literature is clear. I would be delighted to point you toward numerous references. We see no other option if we are to fulfill our mission as teachers.

I look forward to your comments and ideas as we move forward together.

Very truly yours,

Classroom teacher _____

* Again, this is available at SurvivaloftheFit.net.

ACTION LIST FOR REVOLUTIONARIES

Starting a revolution is hard. I talk about the inertia you will face from those in control, but first you must overcome your own inertia. We are all different, but here are some suggestions that might help.

1. Remember your mantra: *"I have more power than I think."*
2. Our present outdated system did not come by divine providence—people—people much like you and I with good intentions—put it there. The sports model was a myth created for the multiple reasons described at the beginning of the 1900s. In truth, it did not serve the majority of children even then, but it was a different world 100 years ago. We cannot rewrite history, but we can write a better future for our youth. Change is needed, and this change can come through our efforts.
3. Build a support group and use them. You will hear a lot of "no's" in this venture. You might even be called some unpleasant names. Some people do not like anyone who rocks the boat—even if it ultimately benefits them and their children. Lean on others. Share the work.
4. Start small. As noted, I settled for a pilot project for just 20 youngsters. Build slowly and collect data (names, numbers, letters of support, etc.) that with time will be impossible to ignore—especially by elected officials.
5. Have goals every week for your action plan—letters to write, meetings to take, beverages to share. Getting something done each week will eventually add up to results, allow you to see accomplishments, and keep your morale high.

6. Stay organized. Establish a Google Classroom, use a whiteboard or bulletin board, whatever it takes to keep things in order. You want to be able to easily see who is responsible for doing what, past and future meeting dates, where letters were sent and when, and so on, so you see progress and continue to move forward.

7. Put pressure on the powers that be to similarly commit to a timeline. When can I expect to hear back from you? When can we meet again to move to the next phase? Who would you suggest I speak with now? Can I tell Ms. Blank this has your support? Be a pit bull and be quantitative. People usually want to do the right thing—they are just unmotivated. You want timelines and action plans, not platitudes.

8. Accept glacial change if need be—but be persistent and do not accept the status quo. If someone has a better idea of how to get us out of this crisis, well, as the Beatles would say, we'd love to see the plan!

TIME AND MONEY

As states go, New Hampshire is on the small size, ranking 46th in the Union. Though it is home to over a million people, when you hear about something happening, you are never surprised when you know the person or recognize the location. To make New Hampshire feel even smaller, if you are a teacher in the state there is an excellent chance you went to Plymouth State University, Keene State College, or the University of New Hampshire, and this makes for a big education family. If any state should be able to be on the forefront of education and educational science, it would be New Hampshire. Yet we are mired in the same ruts as the rest of the country. Despite our size and connections, teachers here are stymied by history, and of course, time and money.

I presented an argument that we can no longer be constrained by history as we live in a new world. I also argued we do have the money, that it was just a question of allocation. Time is a bit tougher. The last I checked we simply are not making more of it. I tried to read Stephen Hawking's *A Brief History of Time* for ideas. I am apparently in the majority of readers who seemingly never quite made it past Chapter 2! The issue of time ultimately boils down to allocation, and I have tried to make the case that PE is where we need more. My goal in this book was to have the reader also appreciate that this should be the case. After almost 40 years as a physician wrestling with the issue of our society's, and especially our children's, decreasing health, I simply see no other viable solution. One of the superintendents I interviewed said, "You cannot legislate your way out of this problem." I would respectfully disagree. Without legislation, without adults working for the common good, just as we did for clean air, clean water, smoking, polio, and dozens of other examples, without action, we will cede the health of the next generation to the computer companies, the sports-industrial complex, and fast food. We are already approaching a "Silent Spring" scenario as children are losing the concept of playing outside. We are better than that. If one school district and then another makes the change to daily, rebranded PE, the state will become healthier. If one state and then another makes the change, America will be healthier. If America changes, other countries will find the impetus to soon follow. And then we will have a true revolution. The "winners"—the average child who does not lose his or her physical identity—will far outpace the "losers": those who perhaps needed to switch from a school-sponsored sport to one that is community based. In the long run, we all benefit from this revolution with smaller medical bills—including those for mental health—a fitter military, a reconnection with nature, higher academic achievement and, I have no doubt, happier children.

My goal in writing *this book* was to introduce numerous positive, available, scientifically based, workable solutions to the present health crisis. I earlier quoted one of my old professors, Rene Dubos, who asked us to "think globally, but act locally." Certainly, this could be the theme for the rebranded PE I suggest. The children we think of as "athletes" are generally those with strong physical identities. We do not have to worry about the health of these youngsters as this identity should continue into adulthood. The children we need to target globally are the vast and increasing majority whose parents and lifestyle do not lend to physical activity. Our job, and to my mind as a physician this is a fairly low bar, should be to get all students to age 18 (starting from the first day of kindergarten) with good health and understanding the benefits of movement. They will then take this knowledge into the rest of their lives because it will be part of their *physical identity*. Graduating a healthy child from high school is the equivalent of graduating with a sixth-grade reading level; that is, it is the least we should be providing for our loved ones. We must raise all boats, not just a privileged few. At high school graduation, there should be an auditorium full of now young adults who have read Toni Morrison *and* know how to perform a squat and hold a plank! As a doctor, I have operated on thousands of people and cared for tens of thousands more. These numbers would be a drop in the bucket as establishing PE for all children, every day, and maintaining their physical identities, would be the greatest health effect I could ever hope to be part of. In the 21st century, the world for our children is indeed *Survival of the Fit*, but it does not have to be a zero-sum game. All children in the world deserve the opportunity to live a long, healthy, and happy life. With all of us working together, we can make that happen. How great is that?

References

Aarts, M.-J., de Vries, S. I., van Oers, H. A. M., & Schuit, A. J. (2012). Outdoor play among children in relation to neighborhood characteristics: A cross-sectional neighborhood observation study. *International Journal of Behavioral Nutrition and Physical Activity*, 9(1), 98.

About SPARK! Spark PE. https://sparkpe.org/about-spark

About Us. (n.d.). Burke Mountain Academy. burkemtnacademy.org/about-us

Ahlskog, J. E., Geda, Y. E., Graff-Radford, N. R., & Petersen, R. C. (2011). Physical exercise as a preventive or disease-modifying treatment of dementia and brain aging. *Mayo Clinical Proceedings*, 86(9), 876–884. www.ncbi.nlm.nih.gov/pubmed/21878600

Aliyari. (2015, July). The effects of FIFA 2015 computer games on changes in cognitive, hormonal and brain waves functions of young men volunteers. *Basic Clinical Neuroscience*, 6(3), 193–201.

Álvarez Bueno, C., Pesce, C., Cavero-Redondo, I., Sánchez-López, M., Garrido-Miguel, M., & Martínez-Vizcaíno, V. (2017, December 1). Academic achievement and physical activity: A meta-analysis. *Pediatrics*, 140(6), e20171498. pediatrics.aappublications.org/content/140/6/e20171498

Alzheimer's Association. (2020). *Causes and risk factors for Alzheimer's disease.* www.alz.org/alzheimers-dementia/what-is-alzheimers/causes-and-risk-factors

American Academy of Pediatrics supports childhood sleep guidelines. (2016, June 13). AAP.org. www.aappublications.org/news/2016/06/13/Sleep061316

American Orthopaedic Society for Sports Medicine. (n.d.). *Youth sports injuries statistics.* Stop sports injuries. www.stopsportsinjuries.org/STOP/Resources/Statistics/STOP/Resources/Statistics.aspx?hkey=24daffdf-5313-4970-a47d-ed621dfc7b9b

Amundsen High School. (n.d.). SchoolDigger. www.schooldigger.com/go/IL/schools/0993000587/school.aspx

Anderson, J. (2018, August 23). *Even teens are worried they spend too much time on their phones.* Quartz. qz.com/1367506/pew-research-teens-worried-they-spend-too-much-time-on-phones

Anderson, L. M. (2006). *"The playground of today is the republic of tomorrow": Social reform and organized recreation in the USA, 1890–1930's.* The encyclopedia of pedagogy and informal education. infed.org/mobi/social-reform-and -organized-recreation-in-the-usa

Anderson, M., & Perrin, A. (2017, May 17). *Technology use among seniors*. Pew Research Center: Internet, Science & Tech. www.pewinternet.org/2017 /05/17/technology-use-among-seniors

Bandura, A. (1977). Self-Efficacy: Toward a unifying theory of behavioral change. *Psychological Review, 84*(2), 191–215.

Begemann, S., Beld, G. V. D., & Tenner, A. (1997). Daylight, artificial light and people in an office environment, overview of visual and biological responses. *International Journal of Industrial Ergonomics, 20*(3), 231–239.

Betts, J. R. (1953, September 1). The technological revolution and the rise of sport, 1850–1900. *The Mississippi Valley Historical Review, 40*(2), 231–256. www.jstor.org/stable/1888926?seq=1#page_scan_tab_contents

Blomain, E. S., Dirhan, D. A., Valentino, M. A., Kim, G. W., & Waldman, S. A. (2013). Mechanisms of weight regain following weight loss. *ISRN Obesity, 2013*, 210524. doi.org/10.1155/2013/210524

Boers, E. (2019). Association of screen time and depression in adolescence. *JAMA Pediatrics, 73*(9), 853–859. jamanetwork.com/journals/jamapediatrics /article-abstract/2737909

Boyce, B. A. (n.d.). *Physical education—Overview, preparation of teachers*. State University.com. education.stateuniversity.com/pages/2324/Physical-Edu cation.html

Brewer, B. W., Van Raalte, J. L., & Lander, D. E. (1993). Athletic identity: Hercules' Achilles heel? *International Journal of Sport Psychology, 24*(2), 237–254.

Burghardt, G. M. (2006). *The genesis of animal play: Testing the limits*. MIT Press.

Busey, C. (2011). Stairs, A. J., Donnell, K. A. (2010). Research on urban teacher learning: Examining contextual factors over time. *Action in Teacher Education, 33*(3), 314–316. https://doi.org/10.1080/01626620.2011.592126

Camire, M., & Trudel, P. (2010, January 25). High school athletes' perspectives on character development through sport participation. *Physical Education and Sport Pedagogy, 15*(2), 193–207. doi.org/10.1080/17408980902877617

Carrera-Bastos, P., Fontes-Villalba, M., O'Keefe, J. H., Lindeberg, S., & Cordain, L. (2011). The western diet and lifestyle and diseases of civilization. *Research Reports in Clinical Cardiology, 2011*(2), 15–35.

Cawley, J., Meyerhoefer, C., & Newhouse, D. (2005, June 13). *The impact of state physical education requirements on youth physical activity and overweight* (NBER Working Paper No. 11411). National Bureau of Economic Research. www.nber.org/papers/w11411

Centers for Disease Control and Prevention (CDC). (2020, April 1). *Adolescent and school health*. www.cdc.gov/healthyyouth/wscc/index.htm

Compulsory education laws: Background. (2016, June 20). Findlaw. https:// education.findlaw.com/education-options/compulsory-education-laws -background.html

Cook, B. (2019, April 19). The slow drip of football's youth participation de-cline continues apace. *Forbes.* www.forbes.com/sites/bobcook/2019/04 /19/the-slow-drip-of-footballs-youth-participation-decline-continues -apace/#2560f84865ce

Council on Communications and Media. (2016, November 1). Media use in school-aged children and adolescents. *Pediatrics, 138*(5), e20162592. pediatrics.aappublications.org/content/138/5/e20162592

DelaPena, C. (2003). Dudley Allen Sargent: Health machines and the ener-gized male body. *Iron Game History, 8*(12), 3–19.

Described and Captioned Media Program. (2011). *CBC National News: Brain gain* [Video]. https://www.youtube.com/watch?v=-nkL6p02FF0

DeSilver, D. (2017, November 30). *How the workforce changed since the Great Recession began.* Pew Research Center. www.pewresearch.org/fact-tank /2017/11/30/5-ways-the-u-s-workforce-has-changed-a-decade-since-the -great-recession-began

Dubos, R. (1977). *The despairing optimist.* The American Scholar.

The Editors of Encyclopaedia Britannica. (2019, September 2). Catha-rine Beecher. *Encyclopaedia Britannica.* www.britannica.com/biography /Catharine-Beecher

Elementary and Secondary Education Act of 1965, as amended by the Every Student Succeeds Act—accountability and state plans. (2016, November 29). www .federalregister.gov/documents/2016/11/29/2016-27985/elementary -and-secondary-education-act-of-1965-as-amended-by-the-every-student -succeeds

Executive Order 13545—President's Council on Fitness, Sports, and Nutrition, 3 CFR 13545 (2010). obamawhitehouse.archives.gov/the-press-office/executive -order-presidents-council-fitness-sports-and-nutrition

Explore Acalanes High School in Lafayette, CA. *GreatSchools.org.* www .greatschools.org/california/lafayette/402-Acalanes-High-School/#Low -income_students

Faigenbaum, A. D., & Bruno, L. E. (2017). A fundamental approach for treating pediatric dynapenia in kids. *ACSM's Health & Fitness Journal, 21*(4), 18–24.

Faigenbaum, A. D., & Macdonald, J. P. (2017). Dynapenia: It's not just for grown-ups anymore. *Acta Paediatrica, 106*(5), 696–697. doi:10.1111/apa.1379

Faigenbaum, A. D., Rebullido, T. R., & Macdonald, J. P. (2018). The unsolved problem of paediatric physical inactivity: It's time for a new perspective. *Acta Paediatrica, 107*(11), 1857–1859.

Farič, N., Yorke, E., Varnes, L., Newby, K., Potts, H. W., Smith, L., . . . Fisher, A. (2019, April–June). Younger adolescents' perceptions of physical ac-tivity, exergaming, and virtual reality: Qualitative intervention develop-ment study. *JMIR Serious Games, 7*(2), e11960. www.ncbi.nlm.nih.gov /pmc/articles/PMC6601253

Fedewa, A. (2011). The effects of physical activity and physical fitness on children's achievement and cognitive outcomes: A meta-analysis. *Research

Quarterly for Exercise and Sport, 82(3). doi:10.5641/027013611x1327519 1444107

Feeney, N. (2014, June 29). 71% of U.S. youth don't qualify for military service, Pentagon says. *Time.* time.com/2938158/youth-fail-to-qualify-military -service

Friedman, H. L. (2013, September 20). When did competitive sports take over American childhood? *The Atlantic.* www.theatlantic.com/education /archive/2013/09/when-did-competitive-sports-take-over-american -childhood/279868

Fu, Y., Burns, R. D., Gomes, E., Savignac, A., & Constantino, N. (2019, August 7). *Trends in sedentary behavior, physical activity, and motivation during a classroom-based active video game program.* www.ncbi.nlm.nih.gov/pubmed /31394855

Gerdy, J. R. (2002). *Sports: The All-American addiction.* University Press of Mississippi.

Gibney, M. J. (2019, February). Ultra-processed foods: Definitions and policy issues. *Current Developments in Nutrition, 3*(2). www.ncbi.nlm.nih.gov/pmc /articles/PMC6389637

Ginsburg, K. R. (2007, January). The importance of play in promoting healthy child development and maintaining strong parent-child bonds. *Pediatrics, 119*(1), 182–191. pediatrics.aappublications.org/content/119/1/182

Gladwell, M. (2009). *Outliers.* Penguin.

Gladwell, M. (2014). *Tipping point.* Little, Brown.

Goldman, D. (2014, January 14). *Does Powerball really fund education?* CNNMoney. money.cnn.com/2016/01/13/news/powerball-education

Greene, J. D., Nystrom, L. E., Engell, A. D., Darley, J. M., & Cohen, J. D. (2004). The neural bases of cognitive conflict and control in moral judgment. *Neuron, 44*(2), 389–400.

Grove, J. R., Lavallee, D., & Gordon, S. (1997). Coping with retirement from sport: The influence of athletic identity. *Journal of Applied Sport Psychology, 9*(2), 191–203.

Harter, S. (1999). *The construction of the self: A developmental perspective.* Guilford Press.

The healthcare costs of obesity. (n.d.). The state of childhood obesity. www.state ofchildhoodobesity.org/healthcare-costs-obesity

Henricks, K., & Embrick, D. G. (2017). *State lotteries: Historical continuity, rearticulations of racism, and American taxation.* Routledge/Taylor & Francis Group.

Hess, A. (2018, January 23). *The 10 most and least educated states in 2018.* CNBC. www.cnbc.com/2018/01/23/the-10-most-and-least-educated-states-in -2018.html

Holderness School: Private boarding & day high school in Plymouth, NH. (n.d.). www.holderness.org

Holland, R. (2018, April). *Where oh where has the Presidential Fitness Council gone?* The Heartland Institute. www.heartland.org/news-opinion/news /where-oh-where-has-the-presidential-fitness-council-gone

How to become a phys ed teacher. (n.d.). www.peteacheredu.org

Hyman, M. (2009). *Until it hurts: America's obsession with youth sports and how it harms our kids.* Beacon Press.

Hyman, M. (2012). *The most expensive game in town: The rising cost of youth sports and the toll on today's families.* Beacon Press.

Illinois State Board of Education. (2012). *Illinois enhanced physical education strategic plan.* www.isbe.net/Documents/epe-strategic-plan0812.pdf

Immigration in the early 1900s. (n.d.). www.eyewitnesstohistory.com /snpim1.htm.

Institute of Medicine. (2013). *Educating the student body: Taking physical activity and physical education to school.* The National Academies Press. doi.org/10 .17226/18314

Jensen, E. (2008). *Enriching the brain: How to maximize every learner's potential.* Jossey-Bass.

John Dewey. (2020, June 15). www.biography.com/scholar/john-dewey

John F. Kennedy Library and Museum. (n.d.). *The federal government takes on physical fitness.* www.jfklibrary.org/learn/about-jfk/jfk-in-history/physical -fitness

Kalish, M., Banco, L., Burke, G., & Lapidus, G. (2010, October). Outdoor play: A survey of parent's perceptions of their child's safety. *The Journal of Trauma, 69*(4 Suppl), S218–S222. www.ncbi.nlm.nih.gov/pubmed /20938312

Kennedy, John F. (1963, August 13). *Progress report by the president on physical fitness.* The American Presidency Project. www.presidency.ucsb.edu /documents/progress-report-the-president-physical-fitness

Kimbro, R. T., & Schachter, A. (2011, October). Neighborhood poverty and maternal fears of children's outdoor play. *Family Relations, 60*(4), 461–475. www.ncbi.nlm.nih.gov/pmc/articles/PMC3172153

Kramer, K. L., & Codding, B. F. (1970, December 1). *Hunters and gatherers in the twenty-first century.* School for Advanced Research. sarweb.org

Krug, E. A. (1969). *The shaping of the American high school, 1880–1920.* University of Wisconsin Press.

Larmer, J. (2016, March 28). *Gold standard PBL: Student voice & choice.* PBLWorks. https://www.pblworks.org/blog/gold-standard-pbl-student-voice-choice

Leahy, R. L. (1985). *The development of the self.* Academic Press.

LeCorre, E. (2018, October 23). *Physical fitness: Its history, evolution, and future.* The Art of Manliness. www.artofmanliness.com/articles/the-history-of -physical-fitness

Lewis, K. P., & Barton, R. A. (2004). Playing for keeps. *Human Nature, 15*(1), 5–21.

Library of Congress. (n.d.). *Rise of industrial America, 1876–1900*. www.loc.gov /teachers/classroommaterials/presentationsandactivities/presentations /timeline/riseind

Ludwig, D. (2017, January 21). *Declining life expectancy according to new CDC data*. Medium. medium.com/@davidludwigmd/declining-life-expectancy -according-to-new-cdc-data-d137ae07d1bb

Maguire, J. (2006). *Power and global sport: Zones of prestige, emulation, and resistance*. Routledge.

Masic, I., Miokovic, M., & Muhamedagic, B. (2008). Evidence based medicine— New approaches and challenges. *Acta Informatica Medica, 16*(4), 219–225.

Massachusetts Department of Education. (1999). *Massachusetts comprehensive health curriculum framework*. www.doe.mass.edu/frameworks/health/1999 /1099.pdf

McMurrer, J. (2008, February 20). Center on Education Policy. www.cep-dc .org/displayDocument.cfm?DocumentID=309

Menand, L. (2019, August 26). The looking glass. *The New Yorker*, 81.

Merkel, D. L. (2013, May 31). Youth sport: Positive and negative impact on young athletes. *Open Access Journal of Sports Medicine*, Dove Medical Press. www.ncbi.nlm.nih.gov/pmc/articles/PMC3871410

Merriam-Webster. (1989). *The new Merriam-Webster dictionary*. Myth.

Miller, G. (n.d.). Failed fitness history. *Kids failed fitness*. www.kidsfailedfitness .org/index.php/failed-fitness-history

Miner, J. W. (2019, April 21). Why 70 percent of kids quit sports by age 13. *The Washington Post*, WP Company. www.washingtonpost.com/news/parenting /wp/2016/06/01/why-70-percent-of-kids-quit-sports-by-age-13

Miracle, A. W., & Rees, C. R. (1994). *Lessons of the locker room: The myth of school sports*. Prometheus Books.

Mississippi Department of Education. (n.d.). *2013–2014 Mississippi Physical Education Framework*. www.mdek12.org/sites/default/files/documents /OHS/health-education-framework_1.pdf

National Association for Sport and Physical Education. (n.d.). www.pgpedia.com/n /national-association-sport-and-physical-education

National Association to Advance Fat Acceptance (NAAFA). (2016). *About NAAFA*. www.naafaonline.com/dev2/about

National Cancer Institute. (2015). *Chronic inflammation*. www.cancer.gov/about -cancer/causes-prevention/risk/chronic-inflammation

National Center for Chronic Disease Prevention and Health Promotion. (2018, September 11). *Childhood overweight and obesity*. Centers for Disease Control and Prevention. www.cdc.gov/obesity/childhood

National Institute of Diabetes and Digestive and Kidney Diseases. (2017). *Overweight & obesity statistics*. www.niddk.nih.gov/health-information/health -statistics/overweight-obesity

Need to Know. (2011, February 8). *A physical education in Naperville* [Video]. PBS. https://www.pbs.org/wnet/need-to-know/video/a-physical-education-in-naperville-ill/7134/

New Hampshire Department of Education. (2005). *New Hampshire K–12 physical education curriculum guidelines.* www.education.nh.gov/sites/g/files/ehbemt326/files/inline-documents/standards-pe.pdf

O'Hanlon, T. P. (1983). School sports as social training: The case of athletics and the crisis of World War I. *Journal of Sport History, 9*(1), 5–29.

O'Neill, D. F. (2008). Injury contagion in alpine ski racing: The effect of injury on teammates' performance. *Journal of Clinical Sport Psychology, 2*(3), 278–292.

O'Neill, D. F. (2008). *Knee surgery: The essential guide to total knee recovery.* St. Martins Griffin.

O'Neill, D. F. (2012). The psychology of the aging athlete. In A. Chen (Ed.), *Orthopaedic care of the mature athlete* (pp. 155–163). American Academy of Orthopaedic Surgeons.

O'Neill, D. F., & Marsden, C. (2017). *The effect of multiple object tracking training on confidence and performance.* Publication pending.

O'Neill, D. F., & Thomas, C. W. (2014). Less is more: Limiting narcotic prescription quantities for common orthopedic procedures. *The Physician and Sportsmedicine, 42*(4), 100–105.

Park, M., Kim, Y. J., Kim, D. J., & Choi, J. (2017, September). Sustained dysfunctional information processing in patients with internet gaming disorder. *Medicine, 96*(36), e7995.

Partridge, J. (2015, February 11). *The role of friendships in youth sports.* National Alliance for Youth Sports. www.nays.org/blog/the-role-of-friendships-in-youth-sports

Pate, R. R., Trost, S. G., Levin, S., & Dowda, M. (2000, September). Sports participation and health-related behaviors among US youth. *Archives of Pediatrics & Adolescent Medicine, 154*(9), 904–911. www.ncbi.nlm.nih.gov/pubmed/10980794

PE4life. (n.d.). Play and Playground Encyclopedia. www.pgpedia.com/p/pe4life

Physical education model content standards for California Public Schools, kindergarten through grade twelve. (2005). www.cde.ca.gov/be/st/ss/documents/pestandards.pdf

Pratt, L. A., & Brody, D. J. (2014, October). Depression and obesity in the U.S. adult household population, 2005–2010. *NCHS Data Brief, 167*, 1–8. www.ncbi.nlm.nih.gov/pubmed/25321386

Presidential Youth Fitness Program. (n.d.). *About us.* pyfp.org

Prince, H., Allin, L., Sandseter, E. B. H., & Ärlemalm-Hagsér, E. (2013). Outdoor play and learning in early childhood from different cultural perspectives. *Journal of Adventure Education and Outdoor Learning, 13*(3), 183–188. doi.org/10.1080/14729679.2013.813745

Pruter, R. (2013). *The rise of American high school sports and the search for control: 1880–1930.* Syracuse University Press.

Pujol, J., Fenoll, R., Forns, J., Harrison, B. J., Martínez-Vilavella, G., Macià, D., . . . Sunyer, J. (2016). Video gaming in school children: How much is enough? *Annals of Neurology, 80*(3), 424–433.

Purcell, L. (2005). Sport readiness in children and youth. *Paediatrics & Child Health, 10*(6), 343–344.

Ransom, M. R., & Ransom, T. (2018). Do high school sports build or reveal character? Bounding causal estimates of sports participation. *Economics of Education Review, 64,* 75–89.

Rasberry, C. N., Lee, S. M., Leah, R., Laris, B. A., Russell, L. A., Coyle, K. K., & Nihiser, A. T. (2011, June). The association between school-based physical activity, including physical education, and academic performance: A systematic review of the literature. *Preventive Medicine, 52*(Suppl 1), S10–S20. www.ncbi.nlm.nih.gov/pubmed/21291905

Ratey, J. J. (2013). *Spark: The revolutionary new science of exercise and the brain.* Little, Brown.

Ratey, J. J., Manning, R., & Perlmutter, D. (2014). *Go wild: Free your body and mind from the afflictions of civilization.* Little, Brown.

Reynolds, G. (2011, August 10). *For better grades, try gym class.* well.blogs.nytimes .com/2011/08/10/how-gym-class-can-help-students-excel

Reynolds, G. (2019, October 2). Being young, active and physically fit may be very good for your brain. *The New York Times.* www.nytimes.com/2019 /10/02/well/move/being-young-active-and-physically-fit-may-be-very -good-for-your-brain.html?searchResultPosition=1

Riess, S. A. (1995). *Sport in industrial America: 1850–1920.* Harlan Davidson.

Riess, S. A. (2011). *Sports in America: From colonial times to the twenty-first century: An encyclopedia.* Sharpe Reference.

Robert Wood Johnson Foundation. (2019). *Physical inactivity in the United States.* The State of Childhood Obesity. stateofchildhoodobesity.org/physical -inactivity

Sack, H. (2018, February 19). *René Dubos and the antibiotics.* scihi.org/rene-dubos -antibiotics

Sattelmair, J., & Ratey, J. (2009). Physically active play and cognition an academic matter. *American Journal of Play, 1*(3), 365–374. johnratey.typepad .com/SattelRatey.pdf

School Breakfast Program (SBP). (n.d.). Retrieved August 21, 2019, from http:// www.feedingamerica.org/take-action/advocate/federal-hunger-relief -programs/school-breakfast-program.html

Serino, L. (2017, April 6). *What international test scores reveal about American education.* www.brookings.edu/blog/brown-center-chalkboard/2017/04/07 /what-international-test-scores-reveal-about-american-education

SHAPE America Society of Health and Physical Educators. (n.d.). *Physical educa-tion guidelines.* www.shapeamerica.org/standards/guidelines/peguidelines.aspx

Slawson, D. J. (2005). *The Department of Education battle, 1918–1932: Public schools, Catholic schools, and the social order.* University of Notre Dame Press.

State Board of Education adopts new physical education, health standards for Iowa schools. (2019, March 28). Iowa Department of Education. educateiowa.gov/article/2019/03/28/state-board-education-adopts-new-physical-education-health-standards-iowa-schools

Swanson, B. (2017, June). *Youth sports participation by the numbers.* ACTIVE-kids. www.activekids.com/football/articles/youth-sports-participation-by-the-numbers

Szabo-Reed, A. N., Willis, E. A., Lee, J., Hillman, C. H., Washburn, R. A., & Donnelly, J. E. (2019, June 15). The influence of classroom physical activity participation and time on task on academic achievement. *Translational Journal of the ACSM, 4*(2), 84–95. www.ncbi.nlm.nih.gov/pubmed/31576376

Taubes, Gary. (2018). *The case against sugar.* Portobello Books.

Teach for America. (n.d.). www.teachforamerica.org

Theisen, E. (n.d.). How America can get physically tough. Physical fitness: A report of progress. *Look.* http://www.loc.gov/pictures/item/2016716140/

Tsang, S. K. M., Hui, E. K. P., & Law, B. C. M. (2012). Positive identity as a positive youth development construct: A conceptual review. *The Scientific World Journal, 2012,* Article ID 529691,1–8.

Union of Concerned Scientists. (2018, January 9). *Scientists agree: Global warming is happening and humans are the primary cause.* www.ucsusa.org/resources/global-warming-happening-and-humans-are-primary-cause

Welcome La Sierra H.S. Longhorns! (n.d.). http://lasierraonline.com

What is CrossFit? (n.d.). www.crossfit.com/what-is-crossfit

What is exergaming? (n.d.). HealthySD.gov. healthysd.gov/what-is-exergaming-5

Williams, F. (2017). *The nature fix.* Norton.

Wilson, E. O. (2003). *Biophilia.* Harvard University Press.

Wooden, J., & Jamison, S. (2018). *The essential Wooden: A lifetime of lessons on leaders and leadership.* McGraw-Hill Education.

Zientarski, P. (2015, May 26). *Want smarter, healthier kids? Try physical education!* TEDxBend. www.youtube.com/watch?v=V81cO8xyMaI

Index

About the Author

Daniel Fulham O'Neill, MD, EdD, is a board-certified orthopedic surgeon and the author of numerous articles in scholarly journals and mass market publications. He is also the author of *Knee Surgery: The Essential Guide to Total Knee Recovery* (2008).

After completing a chemistry degree at Bard College, Dr. O'Neill attended the School of Medicine at the State University of New York at Stony Brook. He performed his surgical training in New York City, Stony Brook, and Eugene, Oregon. Fifteen years into his medical career, he realized a significant part of his practice as a sports medicine doctor and surgeon was the psychological health of his patients. He returned to school and received a doctorate of education (EdD) with an emphasis in exercise and sport psychology from Boston University. He is the only orthopedic sports medicine doctor with such a degree. His unique training coupling the "social science" of our cognitive lives, with the "hard science" of our physical lives gave him a new perspective regarding the present health issues of our youth. This education has been supplemented by years of working with young people at amateur and professional athletic events, in training rooms, and off the field, treating physical and psychological issues.

While early in his career Dr. O'Neill's concern was obesity's effect on knees and other weight-bearing joints, he soon realized this was not just a middle-aged problem. Lack of activity is endemic for a large proportion of our youth. Dr. O'Neill's interest in school physical education came especially from observing a widening of the athlete/nonathlete divide, where the students who did not participate in organized sports were engaging in essentially *no physical activity*. In addition to multiple cultural factors (bad food, computers, and the influence of the sports-industrial complex), he believes a significant aspect of this inactivity is the lack of high-level physical education in our schools leading to the loss of what he has coined "physical identity."

Dr. O'Neill is an adjunct professor at Plymouth State University and the University of New Hampshire, and serves as team physician for multiple local schools. He is an orthopedic surgeon with The Alpine Clinic, a division of Littleton Regional Hospital in New Hampshire. Dr. O'Neill is a member of the New Hampshire Orthopaedic Society, the American Academy of Orthopaedic Surgeons, the American Orthopaedic Society for Sports Medicine, and the American College of Sports Medicine.

Dr. O'Neill shares his life in the Lakes Region and White Mountains of New Hampshire with his wife, Patricia, a long-time elementary educator. Along with their dogs, Lenny and Carlos, they can often be found out on the trails hiking, skiing, or cycling.